# MEDICAL ONCOLOGY

**FUNDAMENTAL AND CLINICAL ASPECTS OF INTERNAL MEDICINE**
**A Series of Volumes for the Postgraduate Course**

THE UNIVERSITY OF MIAMI SCHOOL OF MEDICINE
Department of Internal Medicine
Coordinators
Jose S. Bocles, M.D.
William J. Harrington, M.D.


PUBLISHED
CLINICAL RHEUMATOLOGY
John H. Talbott, M.D., Editor

MEDICAL ONCOLOGY
Howard E. Lessner, M.D., Editor

**FUNDAMENTAL AND CLINICAL ASPECTS OF INTERNAL MEDICINE**
A Series of Volumes for the Postgraduate Course

# MEDICAL ONCOLOGY

Edited by Howard E. Lessner, M.D.

THE UNIVERSITY OF MIAMI SCHOOL OF MEDICINE
Department of Oncology
Comprehensive Cancer Center for the State of Florida

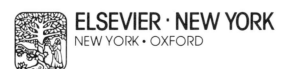

**ELSEVIER · NEW YORK**
NEW YORK • OXFORD

Elsevier North-Holland, Inc.
52 Vanderbilt Avenue, New York, New York 10017

Distributors outside the United States and Canada:
Thomond Books
(A Division of Elsevier/North-Holland Scientific Publishers, Ltd)
P.O. Box 85
Limerick, Ireland

Library of Congress Cataloging in Publication Data

Main entry under title:
    Medical Oncology.

(Fundamental and clinical aspects of internal medicine)
Includes bibliographies and index.
1. Cancer. 2. Oncology. I. Lessner, Howard E. II. Series. [DNLM: 1.
Neoplasms. QZ200 058]
RC261.M468      616.9′94      78-17548
ISBN 0-444-00269-3
ISBN 0-444-00260-X pbk.

MANUFACTURED IN THE UNITED STATES OF AMERICA

DESIGNED BY LORETTA LI

Contributing Authors

NORMAN L. BLOCK, M.D.

LAWRENCE E. BRODER, M.D.

JOHN J. BYRNES, M.D.

KOMANDURI K. N. CHARYULU, M.D.

HOWARD E. LESSNER, M.D.

RICHARD MANN-KAPLAN, M.D.

PETER W. A. MANSELL, M.D.

OLEG S. SELAWRY, M.D.

MICHAEL A. SILVERMAN, M.D.

EVERETT V. SUGARBAKER, M.D.

FRANCISCO TEJADA, M.D.

SHARON THOMSEN, M.D.

MICHAEL B. TRONER, M.D.

CHARLES L. VOGEL, M.D.

C. GORDON ZUBROD, M.D.

# CONTENTS

# GENERAL PREFACE

Four years ago the Department of Internal Medicine of the University of Miami School of Medicine inaugurated an annual series of postgraduate courses entitled "Fundamental and Clinical Aspects of Internal Medicine". The first course, prompted by many requests from area physicians and medical societies, was timed to precede by one to two weeks the initial recertification examination of the American Board of Internal Medicine.

Among the teaching materials developed for this course was a group of booklets designed to follow closely the lecture presentations of subject matter judged to be of most pertinence to internists qualified for certification. Since the course was intensive and of only two weeks duration, we realized that the material to be presented had to be carefully selected, with assumptions made concerning content presumed to be already well known and also concerning material that would not in our judgment be needed by a competent general internist, although of great importance to the subspecialist.

The course has now been given each of the past four years. Its quality has been widely noted, and many physicians both from the United States and other countries have become annual registrants. Accordingly, it was felt that the course booklets might find a wider appeal if they were professionally produced and distributed by a publisher. This objective has been concluded by an agreement with Elsevier North-Holland to publish the series of volumes.

It should be stressed that these volumes are not intended to be comprehensive. They will not cover subject matter in the breadth ordinarily found in standard textbooks, but rather will supplement standard works. In order to be useful for the review course, the books will be inexpensive, and will be updated periodically, to maintain currency with advances in their respective areas.

We acknowledge the immeasurable help of our staff coordinator, Mrs. Arlene Gunn, and the secretarial staff of the divisions who contributed in the preparation of these volumes.

JOSE S. BOCLES, M.D.
WILLIAM J. HARRINGTON, M.D.

# PREFACE TO THIS VOLUME

For several years the faculty at the University of Miami School of Medicine and the Comprehensive Cancer Center for the State of Florida have participated actively in intensive cancer education programs directed at both the undergraduate and graduate levels. This volume is a distillation of these efforts and has been devised to summarize currently important cancer information at the pathological, physiological and clinical levels in a form which we hope will be of value to both medical students and those practitioners who may wish to update their general knowledge in cancer-related subjects. For those wishing to delve deeper into the medical literature, bibliographies have been selected to cover the main points of each chapter.

The format consists of several chapters discussing the pathology and pathophysiology of cancer followed by sections on present general concepts of surgical, radiotherapeutic, chemotherapeutic and immunotherapeutic management. Finally, there are chapters dealing with the pathology, clinical manifestations, prognosis and treatment of some of the more common human tumors.

We trust that this volume will be of help to those faced with the many difficult problems of clinical cancer management.

Howard E. Lessner, M.D.
Professor of Oncology
University of Miami School of Medicine
Clinical Director, Comprehensive Cancer Center
for the State of Florida

# MEDICAL ONCOLOGY

# INTRODUCTORY REMARKS ON THE TREATMENT OF CANCER

C. GORDON ZUBROD, M.D.

As the ability to control some cancers by means of drugs has advanced, the rationale of cancer therapy has been changing, and at this moment the theoretical basis of cancer treatment and its practical application is in the midst of a small revolution. Classic management concentrated on early diagnosis followed by surgical removal, addition of radiation therapy in a few instances, then follow-up to see whether purely local forms of therapy had been curative. The presence of metastatic disease left the physician with nothing to offer except small palliative measures for symptomatic relief and consignment of the patient to a nursing home.

Things began to change with observations in the late 1950s and early 1960s that in two rare tumors—choriocarcinoma and Burkitt's lymphoma—cure of widespread metastatic disease was produced by chemotherapy. By "cure" we mean that some fraction of the treated patients have a normal life expectancy as demonstrated by standard comparison with the life expectancy of the whole population of the same age and sex. Similarly, in a group of nine other neoplasms of children and young adults, normal life expectancy has resulted when drugs were added to surgery or radiation therapy (or both). These potentially curable neoplasms are listed in Table 1 (1).

Although these tumors are for the most part uncommon or rare, it behooves every physician to keep them in mind, because all patients with such diagnoses should have management aimed at giving them their chance at cure.

The list is important in underlining those cancers for which the internist and the pediatrician should be on the alert, and it also serves to introduce the changes that are occurring in the theoretical base underlying the logic of cancer management. All of these drug-sensitive tumors in the list are rapidly growing; that is, they double in volume

## TABLE 1
### *"Cure" Rates in 11 Responsive Cancers*

| TYPE OF CANCER | NORMAL LIFE EXPECTANCY | |
|---|---|---|
| | ESTIMATED % PRIOR TO CHEMOTHERAPY | ESTIMATED % WITH CHEMOTHERAPY |
| Wilms' | 30 | 90 |
| Choriocarcinoma | 20 | 80 |
| Ewing's sarcoma | 10 | 70 |
| Burkitt's lymphoma | 5 | 70 |
| Retinoblastoma | 20 | 55 |
| Acute lympho. leukemia | 0 | 50 |
| Mycosis fungoides | 5 | 50 |
| Rhabdomyosarcoma | 10 | 50 |
| Advanced Hodgkin's | 5 | 40 |
| Diffuse histiocytic lymphoma | 0 | 25 |
| Metastatic embry. testicular | 0 | 10 |

in a matter of days or weeks, whereas tumors such as the common carcinomas that are not so susceptible to drugs are slowly growing, with doubling times measured in months. This difference in growth rate is due to differences in growth fraction or the percentage of cells initiating DNA replication (and subsequent division) per unit time. Thus a tumor with 100% of cells in DNA replication at one moment will grow 10 times faster than a tumor with only 10% of its cells initiating DNA replication. Because most antitumor drugs kill tumor cells when they make DNA (or in a few instances when they divide), a tumor with 100% of its cells making DNA will be totally exposed to the killing capacity of the drug. The tumor with only 10% of its cells in the growth fraction will have 90% of its cells protected from the tumoricidal effects of the drug (2).

It has also been found that the growth fraction is large early in the life history of a tumor. As the tumor ages, the percentage of cells making DNA falls sharply, and thus growth slows with age and drug susceptibility diminishes correspondingly. All of the tumors in Table 1 are discovered when they are young, whereas those of the lungs and gastrointestinal tract are discovered only at quite late stages.

How can this understanding of drug susceptibility as related to tumor age be utilized in reducing the high mortality of the common carcinomas? An experiment of Simpson-Herren (3) and her colleagues provides the clue. In a mouse tumor she examined simultaneously the age and growth fraction of the primary tumor and its metastases, showing that, at a point when the primary tumor had aged and its growth fraction had reduced, the metastatic tumors were young and had high growth fractions. Therapeutic trials by Schabel and his colleagues (4) in a number of mouse tumors have shown that the combination of drugs and surgery gives cure rates much superior to either modality alone. The implication of these studies is that surgery fails because there are occult metastases unaffected by treatment aimed at the local disease. Drugs alone fail because they cure metastases but do not affect the old, drug-insusceptible primary. With the combination, both primary and metastases are eliminated.

Such anticipatory treatment of occult, nondemonstrable metastases following the definitive local removal of the primary cancer has been demonstrated to be effective in a number of clinical situations. Successful combined modality of childhood neoplasms (as shown in Table 1) is well known. In early Hodgkin's disease and in non-Hodgkin's lymphoma the anticipatory treatment is the radiation directed at the total lymph-node areas, where there are nondemonstrable metastases. In acute lymphocytic leukemia success is achieved by chemotherapy of the generalized disease, with local (''prophylactic'') radiation of the whole brain (5). In osteogenic sarcoma, amputation plus intensive chemotherapy has given early indication of prolonged freedom from pulmonary metastases not previously seen from surgery alone. Similarly, in breast cancer with lymph-node involvement in premenopausal women, a 3-year follow-up study showed chemotherapy following radical mastectomy to give far less metastatic relapse than surgery alone.

Recognition of the relationship between cell kinetics and drug sensitivity of tumors has led to the question of whether a solid tumor with few cells in cycle could be stimulated to bring a higher percentage of cells into DNA synthesis, thus rendering the cells susceptible to drugs. Early studies with hormonal stimulation of hormone-dependent tumors did not show a sufficient increase in DNA synthesis to change drug responsiveness. In experimental tumors with few cells in cycle, Schenken and Hageman (6) have shown that after suppression of proliferation following an initial course of chemotherapy there was a recruitment of cells into the proliferative cycle. If a second course of chemotherapy was given at the peak of the proliferative rebound, 90% of the tumors were curable as compared to zero cure rate from the usual intensive chemotherapy. Mauer et al. (7) have applied this reasoning to the design of chemotherapy in children with neuroblastomas. These tumors have generally been relatively insensitive to drugs and few, if any, complete remissions have been achieved in the past. Mauer treated a series of neuroblastoma patients with cyclophosphamide, repeatedly studying the percentage of cells in cycle. Group 1 patients showed a proliferative rebound after cessation of cyclophosphamide, while Group 2 did not. All patients received a course of adriamycin, beginning at the time when Group 1 patients exhibited the proliferative peak. Five of seven Group 1 patients achieved complete remission, while none of the Group 2 patients remitted. This suggests that cells can be recruited into the proliferative, drug-sensitive phases of the cell cycle. Unfortunately, the techniques for determining percentage of cells in cycle are slow and tedious, so that wide study of this principle has not been possible. Recently techniques of cell sorting and flow microfluorometry (FMF) have permitted rapid calculation of the percentage of cells in the various phases of the cycle in the acute leukemias (8). These techniques are being adapted to the so-called solid tumors, which must be broken up to allow study in the flow systems, and it should soon be possible to examine recruitment and its relationship to increased drug effects.

Another way of improving the efficiency of active drugs in human tumors is through pharmacologic manipulation. For example, vincristine alters the permeability of the tumor cell membrane to methotrexate, achieving higher methotrexate concentrations in the tumor. Secondly, methotrexate has been used at relatively low dosage because of its toxicity to normal cells. By means of citrovorum rescue, the normal cells can be protected from much higher doses without any loss of antitumor effect. Both techniques have been used in the highly successful osteosarcoma studies of Jaffe (9) and others. Although this is the only tumor that has been successfully cured to date by these relatively new kinetic and pharmacologic principles, the success of the osteosarcoma studies at least demonstrates the necessity of application of these principles to the common cancers.

# REFERENCES

1. Zubrod CG: Historical perspective of curative chemotherapy. *In* Oncology, 1970. Being the Proceedings of the X International Cancer Congress., Year Book Medical Publishers, Inc., Ed. R.L. Clark, R.W. Cumley, T.E. McCoy, and H.M. Copeland. Chicago, 1971, pp. 337–343.
2. Skipper HS, Schabel FM, Jr: Quantitative and cytokinetic studies in experimental tumor models. *In* Cancer Medicine, Ed. J.F. Holland and E. Frei, III. Lea and Febiger, Philadelphia, 1973, pp. 629–650.
3. Simpson-Herren L, Sanford AH, Holmquisk, JP: Cell population kinetics of transplanted and metastatic Lewis lung carcinoma. Cell and Tissue Kinetics 7: 394, 1974.
4. Schabel FM Jr: Animal models as predictive systems. *In* Cancer Chemotherapy—Fundamental Concepts and Recent Advances. Ed. R.L. Clark. Year Book Medical Publishers, Inc., Chicago, 1975, pp. 323–355.
5. Aur RJA, Simone JV, Husto HO, Vevzosa MS: A comparative study of central nervous system irradiation and intensive chemotherapy early in remission in childhood acute lymphocytic leukemia. Cancer 29: 381, 1972.
6. Schenken LL, Hagemann RF: Recruitment oncotherapy schedules for enhanced efficacy of cycle active agents. Proc Assn Cancer Res 17: 88, 1976.
7. Hayes FA, Green AA, Mauer AM: Correlation of cell kinetic and clinical response to chemotherapy in disseminated neuroblastoma. Cancer Res 37: 3766, 1977.
8. Krishan A, Tatlersall MHN, Paika KD: Flow microfluorometric patterns of human bone marrow and tumor cells in response to cancer chemotherapy. Proc Am Soc Clin Oncol 17: 272, 1976.
9. Jaffe N, Feir E, III, Traggis D, Bishop Y: Adjuvant methotrexate and citrovorum-factor treatment of osteogenic sarcoma. New Engl J Med 291: 994–997, 1974.

# PATHOPHYSIOLOGY OF CANCER AND ITS CLINICAL IMPLICATIONS

JOHN J. BYRNES, M.D.

That the pathophysiology of cancer is as varied as there are patients with cancer is a truism. Nevertheless, some categorizations and phenomenological generalizations may be useful. The pathophysiology of cancer is consequent primarily to the tumor mass and may be either anatomic or metabolic in nature. Anatomic morbidity is a direct result of neoplastic mass invasion and mechanical interference with the function of normal organs. The potential anatomic morbidity is too protean for further elaboration. Metabolic consequences may be due to either consumption of a substance or to production of a substance by the tumor mass. The metabolic aberrations that may ensue are discussed separately under the paraneoplastic syndromes. A consideration of the factors that govern the progression of primary process, the tumor mass, is reviewed; in particular, aspects that pertain to possible clinical intervention are emphasized.

## CELL DIVISION AND REPRODUCTION

### The Cell Cycle

All events of cell reproduction are encompassed within the period called the *cell cycle*. The cell cycle extends from the completion of one cell division to the completion of the next. The cell cycle is divided into four subsections on the basis of chromosome replication and segregation.

The first subsection, which occupies the first part of interphase, is called the $G_1$ (G for growth) phase and extends from the completion of the previous cell division to the beginning of chromosome replication. The beginning of DNA synthesis defines the end of $G_1$ and the

6

initiation of the S (synthesis) phase. The S phase is usually 6–8 hours in mammalian cells and is followed by an interval of usually 2–3 hours, called the $G_2$ phase, which separates the end of chromosome replication, DNA synthesis, from the beginning of prophase in mitosis and cell division. During $G_2$ the various macromolecules are prepared and arranged for the mitotic event. The period of mitosis and cell division is called the M (mitosis) phase and generally lasts less than an hour, returning the cell again into $G_1$.

Whereas $G_1$ is the least well-defined phase of the cell cycle, it is perhaps the most crucial for understanding the regulation and rate of cell replication. The transition of a cell from $G_1$ to S is the critical point in the cell cycle. Once DNA synthesis begins, a cell proceeds quickly to the completion of division and two resultant daughter cells. Thus the decision to divide or not is made in $G_1$. Further, $G_1$ determines the length of the cell cycle as the other phases are fairly fixed in any given cell line. Some rapidly proliferating cells have almost no $G_1$ phase, while other cells (e.g., muscle or neurons) are permanently arrested in $G_1$. That the regulation of the rate at which cells are allowed to reproduce is determined by the retention of cells in the $G_1$ state for a shorter or longer period is shown by the following example. In the alimentary tract of the mouse, the average cell cycle time for the epithelium stem cell varies from 17 hours in the ileum to 36 hours in the colon, to 85 hours for the buccal mucosa to 181 hours in the esophagus. These differences in cell cycle times are due to a change in the duration of only the $G_1$ period of the cycle. The combined duration of the S, $G_2$, and M phases is approximately 10 hours in all cases while the duration of $G_1$ varies from approximately 7 hours in the ileum, 25 hours in the colon, 75 hours for buccal mucosa, to 171 hours in the esophagus (1).

**Tumor Cell Kinetics**

In relating tumor growth to cell proliferation, other factors must be considered, as generally not all the cells in the tumor are proliferating and some cells may be lost. Some nondividing cells are in a sterile vegetative state where they continue to survive but have lost the capability to proliferate. Another type of nondividing cell is in a resting state, retaining the ability to proliferate. Other cells may be restrained from proliferating by a lack of sufficient nutrients. These noncycling cells are referred to as being in $G_0$ (a subphase of $G_1$). The term "growth fraction" is used to indicate the proportion of tumor cells that are proliferating. The growth fraction may be determined by measuring the percent of cells incorporating thymidine over a time period corresponding to the cell cycle length. There is no way histologically to distinguish those cells having the ability to proliferate. Further, all cycling cells are not the same; some have a limited capacity to divide over only several generations. Other cells have the potential to produce an unlimited line of descendants; these are the so-called clonogenic or stem cells. Each cell has the ability to form an isolated clone. Both proliferating cells and cells in $G_0$ state may have clonogenic potential.

Although intermitotic time (cell cycle length) and growth fraction (% cells in cycle) are the major determinants of the input to tumor growth, the output or cell loss factor must be considered to complete the dynamic state. Cells may be lost by a variety of means, including cell death, exfoliation, or migration. Cell death in tumors may be caused by disorganized tissue architecture, with cells unable to receive essential metabolites. Abnormal mitoses may produce cells incapable of survival. Of course, the effect of successful chemotherapy and radiotherapy is to produce cell loss (2).

## FACTORS INVOLVED IN TUMOR GROWTH

### Tumor Angiogenesis and Other Facilatory Factors

Most solid tumors arising spontaneously or from metastasizing cells, or by transplantation in experimental animals, begin as avascular aggregates of malignant cells. The tumor population exchanges nutrients and catabolites with the surrounding interstitial tissue by simple diffusion. This phase of tumor growth is usually microscopic and visible only in a few clinical and experimental situations. Carcinoma *in situ* can be diagnosed in the skin, eye, bladder, and most commonly in the uterine cervix. Carcinomal *in situ* of the cervix may be thought of as a general model for the avascular phase of the majority of carcinomas. In the cervix neoplastic cells may sit superficial to the basement membrane and may remain for years without penetrating it. At some point the membrane is penetrated and almost simultaneously the tumor becomes vascularized. There is a common histological pattern in the skin, pharynx, and gastrointestinal, respiratory, and genitourinary tracts in which the epithelial compartment is separated from blood vessels by a basement membrane. Most carcinomas begin as such and remain small, with growth constraints determined by the process of diffusion.

Rapid growth, and in some tumors exponential growth, starts with vascularization. Vascularization may be responsible for other malignant characteristics of neoplasms in addition to malignant growth. It is possible that metastatic cells may be shed into the circulation only after the onset of vascularization. Circulating tumor antigens may inhibit tumor immunity, and it is possible that antigen pours into the bloodstream only after vascularization. Finally, vascularization may allow for accelerated growth with continued cell proliferation, and malignant characteristics become more prominent with "malignant drift." Tumor angiogenesis is such a point of control because of the peculiarity of solid tumors to stick together. Growing in a packed population, they are subject to the limits of diffusion governing nutrient absorption and catabolite removal. The conditions of the avascular phase are bare survival and population dormancy.

In neoplasia new vessels are induced from the host. Vascular endothelium near the tumor is somehow turned on to migrate toward the tumor implant and to proliferate. A diffusible factor secreted by tumor cells that is mitogenic to vascular endothelium and stimulates capillary proliferation has been partially purified and charcterized by Folkman et al. (3). Tumor angiogenesis factor has been obtained from many malignant experimental and human tumors but is not found in the variety of normal tissues examined. This factor apparently is responsible for the neovascularization of tumor and as such might represent a point for possible intervention with malignant growth. Folkman and colleagues have also demonstrated a diffusible factor from cartilage that inhibits the neovascular growth of tumors (4). When this inhibitory factor is further purified and characterized it may prove useful as a means of maintaining tumor dormancy by *antiangiogenesis*. Clearly, tumor angiogenesis is a critical factor in expediting malignant cell proliferation and growth of solid tumors. A better understanding of this activity and its inhibitors may allow an approach to the control of neoplasia by interruption of its supply lines (5).

The elaboration of lytic substances by neoplastic cells may be equally as important a factor in tumor cell invasion. Neoplastic cell production of hyaluronidase and various proteases has been described (6). Fibrinolytic activity and plasmin activators produced by neoplastic cells in culture have been reported and presumably facilitate tumor spread. Conversely, anticoagulant agents in experimental systems have prevented metastases (15).

## Chalones and Tumor Growth Regulators

Growth regulatory substances have been shown to exist by a variety of observations on normal tissues. Experiments with partial hepatectomy, for example, suggest that the hepatocyte establishes and maintains a specific microenvironment by the continuous addition to the microenvironment of a short-lived repressor that specifically interacts by feedback to inhibit hepatocyte reproduction. The repressor, being short-lived, allows for a rapid proliferative response if its production is decreased by destruction or removal (partial hepatectomy) of its source and regeneration of the organ to the mass that again produced appropriate amount of repressor to then limit its further growth.

The control of cell proliferation by specific and endogenous negative feedback inhibitors of mitosis is the putative function of chalones. The four properties of chalone involve: (1) cell specificity, (2) endogenous origin of the inhibitor, (3) lack of species specificity, and (4) reversibility or lack of cytoxicity. Chalones inhibit the proliferation of cells in $G_1$, and in general a great deal more chalone is required to inhibit a cancer cell than to inhibit the proliferation of a normal cell (8). The fact that neoplastic cells are less sensitive to the effect of chalones may be part of the explanation of mode of growth of cancer cells. As they are less sensitive to the factor that they also endogenously produce, they proliferate to a mass necessary to produce enough chalone to eventually slow their growth. As tumor cells are not insensitive to chalones, their growth is eventually arrested. In addition to other factors, this may explain the low growth fraction commonly observed in some clinical neoplasms. Further, the suppression of the normal counterpart of the neoplastic cell line may likewise be explained by the now excessive production of chalone. Thus, for example, the humoral immunosuppression seen in B-cell neoplasms, or the cytopenias seen with the leukemias and lymphomas that are not on the basis of marrow replacement, may be explained by excessive chalone production by the tumor mass.

The enhanced rate of tumor growth seen in the remainder of a tumor mass when a large bulk is removed may be explained on the basis of chalone production (7). Conceptually, when the tumor mass is large the growth fraction is frequently small due to high chalone production. When tumor is excised, chalone production falls; residual tumor cells are no longer repressed and enter S phase, and so on. Adjuvant chemotherapy about the time of surgery may exploit the increased proliferation of residual tumor as drug sensitivity increases.

### Endocrine Factors and Tumor Growth Control

Hormonal mechanisms are involved in the initiation, progression, and control of many neoplasms. A full discourse on this matter is beyond the scope of this presentation; however, there have been recent advances at the biochemical level that promise to synthesize and condense the current information and observations in this field. The principal function of steroid hormones is the regulation of protein synthesis in the target tissues. After being transported via the bloodstream and penetrating the cell by simple or facilitated diffusion, steroid hormones are bound to specific hormone receptors in the cytoplasm. The hormone receptor complex is then transferred to the nucleus, where it is bound to the target-cell genome. Then by a yet undefined process the target cell responds by increased specific RNA synthesis, followed by increased specific protein synthesis.

All mammalian tissues that require steroid hormones for their optimal growth contain characteristic steroid binding proteins. Thus it is possible to select *a priori* the cancers that will or will not respond to endocrine manipulation. For example, it would appear that human breast cancers fall into two categories, those that contain significant amounts of the estrogen receptor protein and those that do not. These can be distinguished by examination of a cancer specimen *in vitro* (14). In case of metastatic disease most, but not all, patients with receptor-containing tumors will benefit from endocrine therapy. If a cancer shows no distinct evidence of estrogen receptor, that patient has little chance of remission and probably can be spared the trauma of ablative surgery (12).

## DESCRIPTION OF TUMOR GROWTH

### Tumor Growth Kinetics

The simplest means of assessing tumor growth is to make direct serial measurements of tumor size, which can be done in certain experimental and human tumors. Relating tumor weight to time by superficial measurements and using a calibration curve to determine weight provide a "growth curve." Usually with weight plotted vertically (ordinate) and time horizontally (abscissa) on semilogarithmic scales, growth curves are convex upward and flatten out with time (11).

Many attempts have been made to relate a mathematical expression of growth to most situations in order to delineate a past history or predict future growth of a tumor. A modified exponential law of growth (Gompertzian equation) in which successive doublings occur at increasing longer intervals describes the behavior of many tumors. The parameters used are $W_0$, initial tumor size, $A_0$, initial specific growth rate during the observation period, and $\alpha$, the rate of exponential decay of $A_0$. The maximum growth rate occurs when the volume is 37% of the final plateau volume (2).

### Multiple Myeloma as a Model

Multiple myeloma offers a unique opportunity to study the growth kinetics of a human neoplasm. Salmon and coworkers have studied and quantitated the M-component synthetic rate of patients with multiple myeloma and the M-component synthetic rate of their neoplastic plasma cells during *in vitro* culture. Knowing the rate of M-component protein being produced by the patient's tumor mass and the amount secreted by individual cells, they can readily calculate the number of cells that comprise the tumor burden at any time. The unique marker of this disorder thus can be used to determine tumor load and follow its progression or regression. This has allowed the most accurate evaluation of tumor growth and kinetics as has been possible in the human (9).

Recognizing that what pertains to myeloma doesn't necessarily apply to all human neoplasms, and that certain assumptions may not be exact but are a reasonable and best approximation available, then we can obtain some general insight into tumor growth and cell kinetics by studying the myeloma data.

First, it was observed that at clinical presentation there was generally in the range of $10^{12}$ tumor cell burden already present. This range corresponds to about 1 kg of tumor mass. The earliest clinical detectable tumor was $2 \times 10^{10}$ cells, or about 20 g. As myeloma tumor is mostly confined to the bone-marrow space, the lethal limit of tumor mass was about 3 kg, or $3 \times 10^{12}$ cells. Further, the tumor mass at clinical presentation was not rapidly growing; rather, it had a doubling time in the range of several months. This is in contrast to some of the more rapidly proliferating human neoplasms such as the acute leukemias, Burkitt's lymphoma, and choriocarcinomas; however, it is similar to many. Steel (11) measured the doubling time of a variety of human solid tumors and found a range of growth rates extending from periods as short as a week to over a year, with the median in the region of 2 months. A doubling time of 2 months may have several explanations, including rapid proliferation but with excessive cell loss, or just slow proliferation. Generally, and specifically in the case of multiple myeloma slow proliferation is the explanation. Determination of the growth fraction of the tumor is generally less than 5%; thus most of the cells are in $G_0$ at clinical presentation. Following the progression of tumor mass in patients with multiple myeloma confirmed the Gompertzian features to the growth pattern. That is, as the tumor mass became larger there was a slowing of its rate of growth. This was due to cells going out of cycle into $G_0$ with less cells actively proliferating but retaining their clonogenic potential (9).

To accumulate $10^{12}$ cells a clonal origin to multiple myeloma would necessitate 40 doublings of the original cell and its offspring. Thus in all likelihood the doubling time of the tumor wasn't always in the range of months, as this would indicate a preclinical disease of many years. Rather, as an extrapolation of the Gompertzian growth equation back to the origin, and as tumor regression under treatment demonstrates, the smaller the tumor burden, the more rapid the doubling time. Thus the following cell kinetic and tumor growth pattern emerges for this sort of neoplasm. The neoplastic original cell and its daughters double at a maximal rate, cell cycle length being several days and initially all cells in cycle. As the tumor mass accumulates, an increasing percent of cells go out of cycle into $G_0$ (? chalones, ? lack of metabolite), and there is a progressive slowing of doubling time. The preclinical history generated thus is a matter of months rather than years. As the tumor mass enlarges and cells go into $G_0$ they become resistant to the most effective forms of chemotherapy, namely, cycle specific, S-phase specific agents such as Ara C. They are sensitive still to the cycle non-specific agents such as the alkylating drugs and radiation. With a decrease in tumor mass either through chemotherapy, surgery, or radiation, and as one goes down the Gompertzian curve, more cells come into cycle, growth is faster, and apparent resistance to initially effective agents may occur. However, sensitivity to agents that are cycle active may also develop because of the increase in DNA synthesis. Several studies are now featuring consolidation phases that employ cycle-active agents in myeloma patients for this reason.

Generally clinically relevant conclusions that may derive from an understanding of cell kinetics and tumor patterns are:

1. Although chemotherapeutic success has frequently been attained in rapidly proliferating neoplasms by means of cycle active drugs, we must attempt to treat many neoplasms that are actually proliferating more slowly (having a smaller growth fraction) than some normal tissues. Consequently, our most active agents are relatively ineffective, and toxicity supervenes before therapeutic benefit.

2. The fact that many neoplasms grow more slowly than normal host tissues rationalized intermittent high-dose, cell-cycle non-specific chemotherapy. Even if not in cycle, the tumor cells suffer damage as do the normal tissues. However, the normal tissues are able to repair more quickly the damage sustained and are ready to experience another course of chemotherapy at a time when the tumor mass is only partially recovered.

3. As the rate of growth (generally determined by % of cells in cycle) varies according to the tumor mass, there will be a different spectrum of drug sensitivity at low tumor mass versus

high. There may be radical changes after partial resection or otherwise effected decrease in tumor mass. This probably has relevance to the emerging concepts of postsurgical adjuvant chemotherapy and consolidation schemes with cycle-active agents (16,17).

## REFERENCES

1. Prescott DM: Biology of cancer and the cancer cell. Ca 22: 262, 1972.
2. Lightdale C, Lipkin M: Cell division and tumor growth. *In* Cancer 3, Ed. F.F. Becker. Plenum Press, New York, 1975, p. 201.
3. Folkman J: Tumor angiogenesis: Therapeutic implications. NEJM 285: 1132, 1971.
4. Folkman J: Tumor angiogenesis: A possible control point in tumor growth. Ann Intern Med 82: 96, 1975.
5. Folkman J: Tumor angiogenesis. *In* Cancer 3, Ed. F.F. Becker. Plenum Press, New York, 1975, p. 355.
6. Cliffton EE, Angostino D: Factors affecting the development of metastatic cancer: Effect of alterations in clotting mechanisms. Cancer 15: 276, 1962.
7. De Wys WD: Studies correlating the growth rate of a tumor and its metastases and providing evidence for tumor-related systemic growth retarding factors. Cancer Res 32: 374, 379, 1972.
8. Houck JC, Attalah AM: Chalones and cancer. *In* Cancer 3, Ed. F.F. Becker. Plenum Press, New York, 1975, p. 287.
9. Salmon SE: Immunoglobulin synthesis and tumor kinetics of multiple myeloma. Semin Hematol 10: 135, 1973.
10. Schabel FM: The use of tumor growth kinetics in planning "curative" chemotherapy of advanced solid tumors. Cancer Res 29: 2384, 1969.
11. Steel GG: Cytokinetics of neoplasia. *In* Cancer Medicine, Ed. J.F. Holland and E. Frei. Lea and Febiger, Philadelphia, 1973, p. 125.
12. Clifton KH, Sridharan BN: Endocrine factors and tumor growth. *In* Cancer 3, Ed. F.F. Becker. Plenum Press, New York, 1975, p. 249.
13. Wood S, Strauli P: Tumor invasion and metastasis. *In* Cancer Medicine, Ed. J.F. Holland and E. Frei. Lea and Febiger, Philadelphia, 1973, p. 140.
14. Jenson EV: Estrogen binding and clinical response of breast cancer. *In* Cancer Medicine, Ed. J.F. Holland and E. Frei. Lea and Febiger, Philadelphia, 1973, p. 900.
15. Weiss L: A pathobiologic overview of metastases. Seminars Oncol., 4: 5, 1977.
16. Sugarbaker EV, Ketcham AS: Mechanisms and prevention of cancer dissemination. Semin Oncol 4: 19.
17. Block JB, Isacoff JB: Adjuvant chemotherapy in cancer. Semin Oncol 4: 109.

# THE PATHOLOGIST AND HIS APPROACH TO CANCER

SHARON THOMSEN, M.D.

## INTRODUCTION

The pathologic diagnosis of malignant versus benign disease is the major decision the pathologist must make when confronted with a specimen. However, that decision marks just the beginning of the pathologist's job. His responsibility to the patient and clinician is the precise definition of the "cancer" growing in that particular patient at that particular time.

The careful clinical and pathological observations of cancer patients from the times of Hippocrates and Virchow have shown that various cancers behave in diverse ways. The truism that all cancers are not alike has to be a basic tenant in the modern diagnostic and clinical management of the patient with malignant disease. Recent advances in various modes of therapy demand that not only precise histologic classification of the cancer, but also a detailed documentation of the various morphologic manifestations of the host's response to the cancer, are necessary for rational treatment and management. Therefore, in reality the pathologist has to be considered a *pathobiologist*—a student and teacher of the biology of the disease. The diagnosis of "benign" or "malignant" should no longer be acceptable to the clinician. The pathologist's diagnostic reports and discussions with the clinicians have to include the morphologic details reflecting the biology of the cancer as it occurs in a particular patient.

The following discussions illustrate some of the current methods and concepts being studied and used by the pathologist. These discussions are by no means inclusive of all aspects of oncologic pathology, but they do serve to emphasize some areas of current interest.

## METHODS OF MORPHOLOGIC DIAGNOSIS

New techniques and equipment now allow the clinician to enter many orifices and recesses of organs that previously could be reached only by major invasive surgery. These new techniques are productive of cytologic and small biopsy specimens, which can be of great diagnostic importance in the definitive management of the patient. However, the clinician and pathologist have to be acutely aware of the limitations of these techniques.

### Cytology

Needle aspirations of solid tumors and brushing, washing, and scraping of lesions in various viscera, as well as collection of secretions and excretions from various organs, have been productive of cytologic specimens from which diagnoses of cancer have been made. These techniques frequently produce an abundance of cells derived directly from the lesion. However, the cellular smears have limited value. They are not productive of information about the relationships of the cancer with the surrounding tissues. The histologic pattern of the cancer, a feature of great importance in the classification of malignant lymphomas, cannot be determined. Vascular invasion, a prognostically important feature in several visceral cancers, cannot be seen in cytologic smears. The cytologic examination, which in experienced hands is frequently diagnostic of "benign," "suspicious," or "malignant" lesions, nonetheless cannot tell us much about the biology of the patient's disease. The surgeons in some of the large Scandinavian centers routinely perform definitive surgery based on the cytologic diagnoses alone. However, cytologists in most, but not all, medical centers in the United States urge that the diagnosis of the lesion be proven by biopsy prior to the definitive therapy. Fortunately, many of the special techniques to obtain cytological specimens are productive of small biopsies by which the biopsy-proven disease can be determined with one diagnostic procedure.

### Biopsies

Biopsies range from being small bits and pieces of tissue obtained by a biopsy needle or small cutting forceps to excisional biopsies that include the entire lesion. The pathobiologist is limited in his interpretation of the biopsy of the cancer by the type of biopsy he has to study.

Frequently, the small-forceps or needle biopsy can serve only to allow the pathologist to make the diagnosis of the presence or absence of cancer in that piece of tissue. Histologic classification of carcinoma versus sarcoma and the subclassification of carcinomas, especially with the help of special histologic stains, usually is accomplished with the small biopsy. However, unless a fortuitous biopsy is made and *in situ* carcinoma is present or a special differentiated characteristic such as bile production in a hepatoma occurs, the pathologist cannot tell if the carcinoma is primary or metastatic to that organ. Interpretations of biopsies of the liver and lung frequently are complicated by this dilemma. In these cases the pathologist, radiologist, and clinician have to consult each other, pooling their knowledge to delineate the likely possibilities and guide their future diagnostic workup.

Incisional and excisional biopsies usually permit the pathologist to: (1) determine whether the lesion is primary or secondary, (2) precisely classify the lesion histologically, and (3) in the case of the excisional biopsy, determine the lesion size. This latter feature is important in the staging of many carcinomas. Blood-vessel invasion—a feature associated with a poor prognosis for the patient with thyroid, renal, testicular, colon, lung, or breast carcinoma—can be optimally observed in excisional biopsies that allow the pathologist to study the lesion extensively. The local host response to the cancer can best be evaluated in the excisional biopsy.

## IMPORTANCE OF MORPHOLOGIC EVALUATION OF HOST RESPONSE TO CANCER

A major area of investigation is the immune response mounted by the host to his cancer. Considerable evidence is accumulating that the cell-mediated immune response is protective to the host with some types of cancer and may be a major factor in preventing the spread of cancer within the local tissues and to distant organs. On the other hand, the antibody-mediated immune response may actually enhance tumor growth in some human cancers.

Retrospective morphologic studies of mastectomy specimens from patients with breast cancer show that inflammatory infiltrates around veins and within the cancer seem to influence the survival of the patient. Whether these inflammatory cells are associated with the cell-mediated immune response is under investigation at this time. A detailed analysis of the morphology of the lymph nodes draining the organ containing a cancer may be an important factor in predicting the prognosis of the patient. Studies on patients with breast cancer (1,2) and colon cancer (3) have shown that sinus histiocytic hyperplasia in the lymph nodes draining these cancers is a good prognostic sign. The presence of sinus histiocytic hyperplasia, a morphologic reflection of cell-mediated immunity, was associated with fewer lymph-node metastases and a longer survival. Patients who had follicular (germinal center) lymphocytic hyperplasia, morphologic reflection of the antibody-mediated immune response, had a higher incidence of lymph-node metastases at the time of primary diagnosis and shorter survival.

It is to be emphasized that these morphologic studies of the host response have been restrospective and not well correlated with concomitant *in vivo* and *in vitro* immunologic studies. Also, these observations made on patients with breast and colon cancer may not be valid for patients with other types of cancer. Many prospective correlative studies are now in progress in many centers that promise to be productive of a better understanding of the immune and other host responses to tumor growth. The results of these studies will obviously be of importance in the rational choice and application of the various irradiation, chemical, and immunologic therapies available today for cancers.

These incomplete retrospective studies strongly suggest that the pathologist may be able to predict the general biologic behavior of a particular cancer in a particular patient.

The morphological analysis of the local inflammatory response in and around the cancer, the presence or absence of vascular invasion, the morphology of the lymph nodes draining the cancer and the histologic classification and grading of the cancer is important in the evaluation of the patient with malignant disease.

## THE ROLE OF ELECTRON MICROSCOPY
## IN MORPHOLOGIC PATHOLOGY

The transmission electron microscope has allowed the pathologist to peer into the complicated environment of the cytoplasm and nucleus of the normal and diseased cell. Recent advances in scanning electron microscopy have shown significant alteration in cell-surface characteristics of dysplastic and malignant cells that help illustrate much of the biologic behavior of these cells. For instance, dysplastic and malignant transitional epithelial cells in the human urinary bladder have distorted cell-surface structures that seem to be related to the lack of cohesiveness characteristic of malignant cells (4). These observations are of importance of our understanding of the biology of malignant neoplasms, but what is the practical application of the electron microscope to oncologic medicine today?

The electron microscope is valuable in the evaluation of some cancers in which diagnostic morphologic features, such as premelanosomes in malignant melanomas, allow a more precise histologic classification of what seems to be histologically unclassifiable neoplasms at the light-microscopic levels. Tumors of the APUD system frequently are diagnosed correctly only by electron-microscopic demonstration of their cytoplasmic secretory granules (5).

A distressing fact of present medical progress is that the most difficult cancers to classify are the "undifferentiated malignant neoplasms" as observed under the light microscope. These cancers all too frequently are so undifferentiated that examination of the tumor cells by electron microscopy is equally unproductive of illustrating diagnostic morphologic features. However, the value of electron-microscopic evaluation of the morphology of cancer cells cannot be disregarded in these relatively early times of the study of subcelluler morphology of neoplasia. New techniques and accumulation of many observations probably will be productive of new morphologic criteria that will allow the pathologist to better define neoplastic lesions.

It is important for the clinician and pathologist to remember that besides those few cases in which subcellular characteristics allow a more precise histological classification of a cancer, the clinically significant classifications that lead to the selection of the most appropriate therapy are the light-microscopic features of the lesion.

## HISTOCHEMICAL AND IMMUNOLOGIC EVALUATION
## OF MALIGNANT NEOPLASMS

The art and science of histochemical and histoimmunologic studies of cancers have been best developed in the lymphoreticuloendothelial systems. Distinction between poorly differentiated leukemia cells of myelocytic and lymphocytic origin can best be accomplished by use of various histochemical and enzymatic reactions (6).

Demonstration of cytoplasmic granules in "blast" cells that stain with the naphthol-AS-D-chloroacetate esterase (NCA) reaction and Sudan Black is helpful in distinguishing cells of the myelocytic series from cells of the lymphocytic series that do not contain these granules.

Immunofluorescence techniques useful in demonstrating specific antigen and antibodies on the surface and within the cytoplasm of cells have been most successful in characterizing the cell type and function in various lymphoreticular diseases (7,8). The presence of tumor-specific antibody producing lymphocytes and plasma cells in the inflammatory host response to a cancer is presently being evaluated by immunofluorescent techniques in many centers.

Fluorescent histochemical techniques are very useful for specifically identifying the tumor cells of pheochromocytomas and of the APUD system (9–11).

## BIOCHEMICAL STUDIES

Various chemical "markers" of neoplastic disease have been defined and are discussed in detail in another section of this book. The pathologist can use some of these markers to better define the cancer present in a patient.

Patients who have cancers developing in "target organs" of certain steroid hormones such as breast, endometrium, and prostate have cancers containing specific protein "receptors" for these hormones. The presence of these specific receptors in a metastatic adenocarcinoma in a patient with an unknown primary has been proven helpful (10). Not only does the presence of the receptors help to indicate the most likely primary source of the metastatic adenocarcinoma, but it also forms a rational basis of appropriate hormonal therapy for the patient.

## CONCLUSION

Patients no longer have "cancer." They have a definable disease that has a probability of behaving in a predictable biologic fashion and reacting to a specific therapeutic regimen. The pathologist has many resources available to accomplish precise definition of the cancer. He can best do this by having at his disposal the complete clinical data to best interpret what he sees in his microscope and analyses in the laboratory. His interpretation of disease is dependent on the information and tissues given him by the clinician.

> And he will manage the cure best who has foreseen what is to happen from the present state of matters. Thus a man will be the more esteemed to be a good physician, for he will be the better able to treat those aright who can be saved, from having long anticipated everything; and by seeing and announcing beforehand those who will live and those who will die, he will thus escape censure.
>
> From "Prognostics,"
> Hippocrates.

## REFERENCES

1. Black MM: Human breast cancer: A model for cancer immunology. Isr J Med Sci 9:284–99, 1973.
2. Hunter RL et al: Survivor with mammary cancer related to the interaction of germinal center hyperplasia and sinus histiocytosis in axillary and internal mammary lymph nodes. Cancer 36:528–39, 1975.
3. Patt DJ et al: Mesacolic lymph node histology is an important prognostic indicator for patients with carcinoma of the sigmoid colon: An immunomorphologic study. Cancer 35:1388–97, 1975.
4. Weinstein RS: Changes in plasma membrane structure associated with malignant transformation in the human urinary bladder epithelium. Cancer Res 36:2518–24, 1976.
5. Pearse AGE: The APUD cell concept and its implications in pathology. Pathology Annual 9:27–41, 1974.
6. Bennett J et al: Acute leukemia. Cytochemical profile: Diagnostic and clinical implications. Blood Cells 1:101–8, 1975.
7. Braylan RC et al: Malignant lymphomas: Current classifications and new observations. Pathology Annual 10:213–70, 1975.

8. Jaffe ES et al: Nodular lymphoma, evidence for origin from follicular B lymphocytes. New Engl J Med 290:813–20, 1974.

9. DeLellis RA et al: Ultrastructure and *in vitro* growth characteristics of a transplantable rat pheochromocytoma. Cancer 32:227–35, 1973.

10. Golomb HM and Thomsen S: Estrogen receptor: Therapeutic guide in undifferentiated metastatic carcinoma in women. Arch Intern Med 135:942–45, 1975.

11. Pearse AGE et al: Polypeptide hormone production by "carcinoid" apudomas and their relevant cytochemistry. Virchows Arch B Cell Path 16:95–109, 1974.

# PARANEOPLASTIC SYNDROMES

LAWRENCE E. BRODER, M.D.

The effects of malignant disease are usually a result of the replacement of normal tissues by malignant growth. However, numerous syndromes have been described that cannot be explained by simple invasion or replacement of an organ but are felt to be due to remote effects of the tumor. These remote effects are usually referred to as paraneoplastic syndromes and encompass a series of categories, the best known of which are the endocrine–metabolic syndromes (paraendocrine) and the neurogenic–paraneoplastic syndromes. Other categories of paraneoplastic syndromes include perturbation of host physiology, alterations in hematopoesis, changes in blood coagulability, and gastrointestinal cancer syndromes, as well as syndromes associated with the effects cancer treatment per se.

## ENDOCRINE–METABOLIC SYNDROMES

Various endocrine–metabolic abnormalities have been described in the cancer patient and include various systemic effects of tumors, osteoarthropathies, as well as paraendocrine syndromes. Cachexia, protein depletion, glucose depletion, and fluid and electrolyte abnormalities are systemic effects of tumors that are best described as metabolic in nature.

The pathogenesis of anorexia and subsequent weight loss in patients with cancer is still ill-defined. It has been demonstrated that abnormalities of taste sensation may be an important physiologic determinant in the anorexia of malignancy. However, it should be pointed out that the mechanisms resulting in taste abnormalities are not well understood. Some explanations include a decrease in taste-bud renewal, a change in the amount and character of salivation, and the coexistence of possible deficiency states such as zinc deficiency. It has also been postulated that lactate may play a role as an anorexogenic agent. The concomitant weight loss in patients with anorexia is usually first manifested as fat loss. Other possible factors are malabsorption syndromes, which may be related to the chemotherapy itself or by tumor infiltration of the gut, such as in the lymphomas.

Protein depletion (manifested usually as hypoalbuminemia) has been documented in patients harboring tumors. Nitrogen-balance experiments have generally been inconclusive. The rate of albumin synthesis has been demonstrated to be decreased in cancer patients. Certain preclinical studies also indicate that tumor tissue may utilize albumin. The hypoalbuminemia seen in cancer patients has been correlated with the extent of the carcinoma and has been used in clinical trials as a measure of response or progression.

Glucose depletion has been described and may be severe enough to induce nonhyperinsulinemic hypoglycemia. This syndrome is seen in 50% of large fibrosarcomas and in 30% of hepatomas. About 90% of these tumors grow in the retroperitoneal space or the liver. The majority of tumors that exhibit this syndrome have total weights exceeding 1 kg. There have been two postulates to explain the hypoglycemia in these cases: (1) excessive utilization of glucose by the tumor and (2) the elaboration of a substance capable of increasing peripheral glucose utilization. The treatment of the syndrome is massive glucose infusions and hyperalimentation. However, recent studies indicate that hyperalimentation may increase weight but offers very little improvement in overall survival.

Fluid and electrolyte abnormalities have been described in patients with carcinomas. Total body water is consistently elevated in cancer patients and this has been confirmed in tumor-bearing animals. The pathogenesis of this is not clear, but many factors may be interrelated, some of which have been previously described (i.e., hypoalbuminemia). Hyponatremia has been related to the sick-cell syndrome as well as to hyperaldosteronism and the inappropriate ADH syndrome. Many times these syndromes will be concurrent. Hypernatremia has been described in CNS tumors where the patient is unable to respond to thirst stimulation. A general discussion of fluid and electrolyte abnormalities with regard to the inappropriate ADH syndrome and other paraendocrine syndromes are described in more detail below.

## PARAENDOCRINE SYNDROMES

Paraendocrine syndromes result from the elaboration of trophic substances leading target-organ production of hormones or ectopic secretion of the active hormone per se. A number of hormonal syndromes
are associated with tumors of the neural crest and have been described
by several investigators as apudomas. Such tumors include medullary
thyroid carcinomas, oat-cell carcinoma of the lung, pancreatic islet-
cell carcinomas, carcinoid tumors, and other tumors of the argentaffin
cells. The characteristics of ectopic humoral syndromes is that they
are usually polypeptides (except for serotonin), are usually not occult
(except carcinoid), are associated with high levels of hormone production, and exhibit physiological lawlessness. The proof of tumor
production depends on the presence of the hormone in the blood, a
change of hormonal level with removal of tumor or with recurrence,
*in vitro* production by tumor (i.e., the Chago cell line, HCG-producing
cell line), as well as the determination of AV differences in level of
hormone across the tumor.

### Hypertrophic Pulmonary Osteoarthropathy

Certain syndromes are always associated with hormone production,
whereas others are generally less often associated with hormonal levels. One example of the latter is hypertrophic pulmonary osteoarthropathy. The clinical features include clubbing of the fingers with painful
and warm swelling of the joints of the distal extremities. Joint effusions
and synovitis are common, and the diagnosis is made by evidence of
periosteal elevation of the long bones. This syndrome has been associated with isolated reports of elevated growth hormone levels. It is
generally seen in adenocarcinomas of the lung but is also seen in nonmalignant disease such as ulcerative colitis and bronchiectasis. It will
generally respond as the tumor responds to treatment. Other hormonal
syndromes are almost always associated with the elaboration of hormone, and we discuss these in subsequent paragraphs.

### Inappropriate Antidiuretic Hormone Secretion (SIADH)

The inappropriate ADH syndrome (SIADH) has as its primary clinical feature hyponatremia, which is usually associated with weakness, confusion, incoordination, and convulsions, especially when the serum sodium concentration is below 100 meq/liter. The pathophysiology is an increase in the permeability of the distal nephron to water by excessive amounts of ADH. Excessive water consumption is also seen in these individuals. It is most often associated with small-cell carcinoma of the lung but has been seen in other tumors of the neural crest. The diagnosis depends on the demonstration of ADH in extracts of tumor as well as the clinical recognition of a hyperosmolar urine compared to an hypoosmolar serum. In the differential diagnosis one must rule out adrenal insufficiency, but the SIADH syndrome is usually not associated with azotemia, hypotension, or hyperkalemia seen in the former. There are many nonmalignant causes of the syndrome, including pulmonary disease such as tuberculosis and aspergillosis, as well as CNS trauma or infection. The treatment is usually fluid restriction with the use of hypertonic solutions reserved for life-threatening hyponatremia. It will often respond when the tumor is treated; however, it should be pointed out that certain drugs such as Vincristine as well as high-dose Cytoxan will often precipitate this syndrome. Recent reports have indicated some success with treatment with lithium, a well-known inhibitor of vasopressin action, as well as with demechlocycline, another ADH inhibitor.

### Ectopic Adrenocorticotropic Hormone (ACTH)

The ectopic ACTH syndrome is another syndrome associated with the production of a trophic hormone affecting a target organ, in this case ACTH affecting the adrenal gland. The clinical features are similar to other hyperadrenocortical states and include florid complexion, thin skin, hypokalemic alkalosis, and ecchymoses. However, due to the rapid onset and short survival of many patients with the syndrome, one sees less central obesity and cutaneous striae than in other hyperadrenocortical states. The pathophysiology is directly related to high levels of circulating cortisol. It is often seen in the apudoma-type carcinomas such as small-cell carcinoma of the lung, non-$\beta$ islet-cell carcinoma, thymoma, and carcinoid tumors. In most cases the tumor is not occult. In 90% of these cases they usually present with metastatic disease or regionally invasive disease that is nonresectable. The diagnosis depends on the finding of high and nonsuppressable levels of plasma cortisol and ACTH. The onset of symptoms is usually rapid. Definitive diagnosis depends on demonstrating high levels in the tumor or effluent blood. Included in the differential diagnosis are other hyperadrenocortical states and Cushing's syndrome. The treatment of the syndrome, which may be life threatening, is directed at the primary tumor. If the tumor is not resectable and life expectancy is relatively long, one may consider bilateral adrenalectomies with replacement therapy, or medical adrenalectomies with aminoglutethimide or *ortho–para* DDD.

## Ectopic Gonadotropin (HCG)

Precocious puberty in children and gynecomastia in the male are indicative of a syndrome due to elevated gonadotropin levels. In the male, HCG stimulates the gonads to produce estrogens and androgens, and high levels of estradiol secretion have been demonstrated in males harboring HCG-producing tumors. The pathology indicates a coexistence with many types of tumors but ectopically is primarily associated with bronchogenic carcinoma of the large-cell anaplastic carcinoma type. Diagnosis depends on demonstrating high levels of gonadotropin that cannot be suppressed with estrogens or androgens. The differential diagnosis includes the various causes of eutopic hypergonadotropin secretion such as ovarian or testicular tumors. The treatment is again directed against the primary tumor. Because this syndrome is not life-threatening, rapid treatment is generally not as imperative as is in the two previously described syndromes. The levels of gonadotropin may also been used to follow a patient's course in relation to therapy, as has been described for prostatic carcinoma and bronchogenic carcinoma (8,9).

## Ectopic Parathyroid Hormone Secretion (PTH)

In the ectopic parathyroid hormone syndrome, hypercalcemia leading to lethargy, weakness, and nausea and vomiting is the prominent clinical feature. Unlike the eutopic syndrome due to benign parathyroida-denomas, one does not see bone resorption or renal lithiasis. The pathophysiology is explained by the persistent secretion of parathyroid hormone despite the presence of hypercalcemia leading to greater bone resorption and increased gut calcium absorption. Parathyroid hormone secretion also promotes phosphate excretion leading to hypophosphatemia. It is mainly seen in visceral tumors such as lung and pancreas but also has a very high occurrence rate in tumors of the head and neck. The diagnosis depends on the demonstration of hypercalcemia, hypophosphatemia, and a low level of tubular resorption of phosphate. High levels of the hormone have also been demonstrated. The differential diagnosis must rule out other causative factors such as eutopic causes of hypercalcemia, for example, primary hyperparathyroidism. However, in the paraneoplastic syndrome the calcium is usually above 14 mg% and is associated with weight loss and other evidence of chronic disease. The absence of renal lithiasis, bone resorption and a family history should point toward the diagnosis of the paraneoplastic syndrome. The treatment is usually directed toward the primary with the usual supportive care in treating hypercalcemia, such as oral phosphates, saline infusions, and mithramycin or salmon calcitonin.

## Ectopic Thyroid Stimulating Hormone (TSH)

The ectopic thyroid stimulating hormone syndrome (TSH) is due to TSH effect on the thyroid leading to excess thyroid hormone secretion, resulting in weight loss, tachycardia, excessive perspiration, and increases in basal metabolism rate, radioactive thyroidal iodide uptake, and serum thyroxine. The pathophysiology relates to excessive levels of TSH affecting the end organ, the thyroid. It has only been found in placental neoplasia such as choriocarcinoma. The diagnosis depends on demonstrating high levels of $T_3$ and $T_4$ in association with high thyroidal radioactive iodine uptake that cannot be suppressed with thyroid hormone. The differential diagnosis is between toxic adenoma, Grave's disease, and the ectopic TSH syndrome. In the ectopic TSH syndrome the gland is only minimally enlarged, the gland is diffusely enlarged, and there is no long-acting thyroid stimulating activity. The treatment is to treat the primary tumor where methotrexate is quite effective.

## Ectopic Thyrocalcitonin

Ectopic thyrocalcitonin has been described in patients with carcinoma of the lung. Eutopically it has been described in medullary thyroid carcinomas. It is usually not associated with hypocalcemia, and the diagnosis is based on the demonstration of high levels of thyrocalcitonin in the blood. The pathophysiology is explained by the secretion of thyrocalcitonin either by the parafollicular cells of the thyroid as an effect of the tumor or ectopically produced by the tumor itself. It is seen in medullary carcinoma of the thyroid and small-cell carcinoma of the lung and has also been responsive in breast tumors. The diagnosis depends on the demonstration by radioimmunoassay of elevated thyrocalcitonin in the serum. Differential diagnosis is between medullary carcinoma, bronchogenic carcinoma, bone metastases, and Sipple's syndrome. The treatment is directed at the primary tumor. Serial calcitonin measurements may reflect the effectiveness of treatment measures.

## Hypoglycemia and Hyperinsulinism

Spontaneous hypoglycemia may be due to dysfunction of endocrine glands but more often than not results from breakdown of metabolic processes regulating glucose homeostasis. At least 100 different disease categories have been known to cause the hypoglycemia, which includes overaction of insulin, liver disease, endocrine disorders, functional nervous disease, chronic barbiturate addiction, pregnancy and lactation, leucine, fructose and galactose sensitivity, and nonpancreatic neoplasms. In a prior section a discussion of nonhyperinsulinemic hypoglycemia concentrated on the glucose depletion seen in very large retroperitoneal tumors. This section discusses the various causes of hypoglycemia related to the hypersecretion of insulin with specific emphasis on benign and malignant pancreatic islet-cell tumors.

The correlation between the extent of hypoglycemia and severity of the symptoms it produces is poor. For this reason, the various conditions are usually grouped under the heading of neuroglycopenia, since the primary symptom of hypoglycemia involves processes of mentation and consciousness. Furthermore, the symptoms must be correlated with the documentation of chemical hypoglemia (blood glucose < 40 mg% or plasma glucose < 45 mg%) and should be relieved with intravenous glucose.

In the adult three syndromes of neuroglycopenia are recognized. The first is acute neuroglycopenia, which affects the autonomic nervous system leading to a vague sense of panic, ill health, and anxiety with palpitations, restlessness, nausea, tachycardia, facial flushing, and sweating. This is usually associated with an overdose of insulin or other causes of severe hyperinsulinism such as pancreatic islet-cell tumors. Subacute neuroglycopenia is characterized by lethargy, somnolence, reduced activity, and stupor. This is usually secondary to prolonged states of hypoglycemia that are unrecognized. Chronic neuroglycopenia is fairly rare, and its onset is insidious, leading to defective memory, psychoses, and paranoia. Other signs of hypoglycemia include diplopia, strabismus, and transient hemiparesis, which are all reversed by glucose infusion.

For practical purposes spontaneous hypoglycemia due to abnormal insulin secretion can be further subclassified into fasting hypoglycemia, stimulative hypoglycemia, and fasting and stimulative hypoglycemia. Fasting hypoglycemia is almost always due to hyperinsulinism from either a benign or malignant insulinoma, islet-cell adenomatosis, islet-cell hyperplasia or non-$\beta$-cell neoplasms that secrete a hormone with insulin-like activity. The stimulative hypoglycemias are usually subcategorized as reactive hypoglycemia and include tachyalimentation (postgastrectomy syndrome), reactive functional hypoglycemia, and reactive hypoglycemia secondary to diabetes. The fasting and stimulative hypoglycemias are seen in idiopathic familial hypoglycemia such as McQuarrie's syndrome or leucine sensitivity.

The fasting and stimulative hypoglycemia subcategorized as idopathic familial hypoglycemia is seen primarily in infants during the first 2 years of life. Eighty-nine percent of these patients have a family history of diabetes, and if one examines the relatives, the presence of abnormal glucose tolerance can be determined. Hypernormal levels of immunoreactive insulin are seen (leucine increases immunoreactive insulin), and one also notes decreased hepatic gluconeogenesis. The clinical features are fasting hypoglycemia primarily after leucine injection with the subsequent neurological sequelae. The diagnosis is made primarily by either an overnight fast or 48-hour fast leading to hypoglycemia, and especially by the leucine tolerance test. The glucagon test is only of moderate importance. The fasting insulin level should indicate hyperinsulinism. The 5-hour glucose tolerance test (GTT) is equivocal. The treatment of this condition includes frequent feedings, steroids, epinephrine, subtotal pancreatectomy, zinc glucagon, or diazoxide, all of which are maneuvers designed to increase glucose levels in the blood. Some patients have a spontaneous remission by 6–10 years.

Stimulative hypoglycemia subcategorized as tachyalimentation occurs in 1–44% of postgastrectomy patients. It is less common after Bilroth II procedures than Bilroth I procedures. It is a late component of the dumping syndrome usually beginning after 2–3 hours. Hypersecretion of insulin in response to high and prolonged hyperglycemia versus activation by glucose of intestinal hormones that stimulate insulin secretion such as glucagon and secretin are included in the etiology. The clinical features include hyperglycemia 2–3 hours after ingestion of a carbohydrate meal and may or may not be preceded by dumping in postgastrectomy patients. The clinical features are usually acute neuroglycopenia. The diagnosis is usually based on fasting normoglycemia and a significant and marked apogee on the oral GTT (hyperglycemia) followed by a hypoglycemic response that occurs typically at 2 hours after glucose administration. The treatment includes frequent feedings of a high-protein, high-fat, and low-carbohydrate diet. Anticholinergics have also been utilized.

The reactive functional hyperglycemia is another subcategory of stimulative hypoglycemia and is the most common type of spontaneous hypoglycemia described. The etiology is somewhat unclear, and one group of patients have demonstrated hyperinsulinism due to possible CNS stimulation. Other features include hyperresponse to glucagon indirectly or directly. Some have also postulated a decrease and sensitivity to glucagon. The clinical features include hypoglycemia 2–4 hours after a carbohydrate meal in an anxious, tense, conscientious, and obese patient. The clinical features are of acute neuroglycopenia. The diagnosis depends on fasting normoglycemia and hypoglycemia and neuroglycopenia 3–4 hours after the oral GTT test, which may or may not show concomitant hyperinsulinism. The treatment is to correct the emotional instability and frequent feedings of a high-protein, high-fat, and low-carbohydrate diet.

The third category of stimulative hypoglycemia includes the subcategory reactive secondary to diabetes. This is usually seen in early chemical diabetes, and the etiology is a delay but exaggerated response in insulin secretion following hyperglycemia after a glucose load. The clinical features include hyperglycemia 3–5 hours after a carbohydrate meal, and it is usually manifested as acute neuroglycopenia. The diagnosis is made by demonstrating a blood glucose that shows a hypernormal apogee with a very slow return to normal (1 hour > 160, 2 hours > 120) with a sudden fall between 3–5 hours. Insulin levels show a slow rise to hypernormal levels with a much slower decline. Patients with this disease usually have normal or slightly elevated fasting blood sugars. The treatment is oral hypoglycemics if one sees a failure to respond to weight reduction and dietary manipulations.

The last category to be discussed in detail is fasting hypoglycemia. In fasting hypoglycemia one must rule out chronic pancreatitis, idiopathic and/or leucine sensitivity primarily in the pediatric age group, fructose sensitivity, and other endocrinopathies before entertaining the diagnosis of insulinoma. Other well-recognized endocrine diseases that can cause fasting hypoglycemia include partial or total panhypopituitarism, adrenocortical insufficiency, and selective deficiencies of growth hormone, ACTH, or glucagon. Insulinoma, however, is unique, in that hyperinsulinism is the cardinal feature of the diagnostic workup.

A study of islet-cell adenomas has elucidated to a great extent the biosynthesis of insulin itself. The existence of proinsulin, the single polypeptide chain precursor of insulin, was first demonstrated in studies of insulin biosynthesis in human islet-cell adenomas. When slices of these tumors were incubated with labeled amino acids, radioactivity was first incorporated in a protein of higher molecular weight which was, however, immunologically related to insulin. It consisted of the A and B chains of insulin linked by an additional polypeptide segment now called the C chain.

It is now clear that the primary structure of proinsulin determines the characteristic tertiary structure and the necessary alignment for the disulfide bonding, that stabilizes the molecule. The proinsulin molecule (mol. wt. 9000) begins with an aminoacid sequence of the B chain at the N terminus and continues through a connecting segment, the C-peptide, (mol. wt. 3000) and terminates with the aminoacid sequence of the A chain. The C-peptide is selectively removed within the $\beta$ cell leaving the two chains, now joined only by the disulfide bonds of the insulin molecule (mol. wt. 6000). The C-peptide is retained within the granules and eventually secreted into the circulation along with insulin in equivalent amounts. The amount of proinsulin within the pancreas is about 1.6% of total insulin, although much larger quantities have been found in human islet-cell tumors (< 52%), suggesting a defect in the enzyme response for deleting the C-peptide. No other specific function has been proposed for the C-peptide. Other comparative properties of insulin and proinsulin include the same crystallization pattern, the fact that proinsulin is immunologically 50% as active as insulin, a biological activity which is from 65% to 98% in the fat-cell assay and the rat diaphragm assay, and that proinsulin represents only 5–20% of total circulating insulin molecule. The presence of proinsulin as a contaminant in the insulin assay may not be of significance in normal subjects, but it may be a dominant feature in patients with insulinomas. It also may be responsible for the antibodies that appear in patients treated with insulin.

Hyperinsulinism due to insulinoma is a fairly rare condition with an incidence of less than 0.6% of all malignant disease from data of the Connecticut Cancer Tumor Registry. Ninety percent of insulinomas are benign adenomas, while 10% are malignant and occur primarily at age 35–55 years, with a predominance of malignant disease seen in the older age groups. With regard to the etiology, 3% usually have had preexisting diabetes, and a family history of diabetes can be elicited in 25–35% of cases. There is a frequent association with multiple endocrinomatosis. The clinical features include subacute neuroglycopenia, usually of insidious onset. Sixty percent of the hypoglycemia episodes occur in the morning. Patients with malignant disease demonstrate the most severe hypoglycemia. The diagnosis can be made with fairly high certainty by the 48-hour fast and a tolbutamide or glucagon-tolerance test. The leucine tolerance test is only marginally useful, and the 5-hour GTT is generally not very diagnostic. The fasting insulin levels may vary and are in general not very helpful, except during an episode of an acute attack. Arteriography in this disease indicates a tumor that is quite vascular in contradistinction to adenocarcinoma, which is relatively avascular. The primary treatment of this disease is pancreatectomy in either benign or malignant stage. Unfortunately, some of these tumors are multicentric and may be metastatic. Frequent feedings with utilizable carbohydrate and glucose and glucagon for the acute episodes are advised. Diazoxide is usually used for maintenance in the unresectable cases. In metastatic malignant insulinoma, which is described next, Streptozotocin is the treatment of choice.

Between 1968 and 1972, 52 patients with metastatic pancreatic islet-cell carcinoma were evaluated for clinical features and response to therapy with streptozotocin (5,6). Seventy-nine percent of the patients had functioning tumors with the majority secreting insulin, and 21% had nonfunctioning tumors. The tumors were found primarily in the tail or pancreas and were noted with equal frequency in men and women at a median age of 52 years. Metastases were mainly to the liver and by local extension, whereas distant metastases were rarely noted. The most frequent presenting symptom was hypoglycemia, occurring in 90% of the functional tumor patients. Gastrointestinal ulceration and diarrhea were less frequently observed. Several patients demonstrated the secretion of several hormones in addition to insulin, including ACTH, gastrin, and glucagon. An overall median survival of 908 days from diagnosis to last follow-up was noted, indicating a disease of a low degree of malignant potential. There was no significant difference in survival rate between the sexes or between the functioning as compared to the nonfunctioning tumor patients (see Table 1).

The treatment of choice in metastatic pancreatic islet-cell carcinoma is Streptozotocin. The clinical experience with Streptozotocin as in these 52 patients with metastatic islet-cell carcinoma was analyzed. The drug was given intravenously in 44 patients and intraarterially in eight (most often on a weekly schedule of administration or 0.6–1.0 g/m²2 IV body surface area). Biochemical responses were seen in 64% of evaluable functional cases, and measurable disease responses were seen in 50% of these cases. Insulin responses occurred 2–3 weeks after drug administration at a total dose of 2–4 g/m² body surface area. A significant increase in one-year survival rate and a doubling of median survival were shown for the responders as compared with the nonresponders. Acute toxicity, consisting of nausea and vomiting, was observed in 98% of the cases, whereas renal or hepatic toxicity was seen in 65% and 67% of the cases, respectively. Hematological toxicity, observed in 20% of the cases, was mild. Renal and hepatic toxicity were usually reversible, but five patients died in renal failure.

**TABLE 1**

*Characteristics of Metastatic Islet-cell Carcinoma Patients*
*Treated with Streptozotocin (5,6)*

| DATA | PATIENTS WITH FUNCTIONAL TUMORS | | PATIENTS WITH NONFUNCTIONAL TUMORS | |
|---|---|---|---|---|
| | NO. | % | NO. | % |
| Pretreatment hormone excretion | | | | |
| ↑ Insulin | 26/35 | 74 | | |
| ↑ Gastrin | 1/35 | 3 | | |
| ↑ ACTH, cortisol, or both | 2/35 | 6 | | |
| ↑ Insulin + gastrin | 2/35 | 6 | | |
| ↑ Insulin + glucagon | 2/35 | 6 | | |
| ↑ Insulin + glucagon + gastrin | 1/35 | 3 | | |
| Insulin normal | 1/35 | 3 | | |
| Presenting symptoms | | | | |
| Hypoglycemia | 37/41 | 90 | | |
| Gastrointestinal ulceration | 6/41 | 14 | 1/7 | 14 |
| Diarrhea | 4/41 | 10 | 1/7 | 14 |
| Diabetes | 1/41 | 2 | | |
| Abdominal pain | 2/41 | 4 | 2/7 | 28 |
| Abdominal mass | 0/41 | | 1/7 | 14 |
| Melena | | | 1/7 | 14 |
| Fever | | | 1/7 | 14 |

## NEUROGENIC PARANEOPLASTIC SYNDROMES

Metastatic involvement by tumor is the most common neurologic complication of cancer. However, the diagnosis of the remote effects of cancer on the nervous system may be made once a direct effect is ruled out. Chemotherapy per se can cause peripheral neuropathy or myopathies such as with Vincristine in the former and by steroids in the latter. The reported incidence of neurogenic complications varies between 5% and 10%.

Nonmetastatic neurologic involvement can be divided into several categories such as encephalopathies, myelopathies, peripheral neuropathies, and myopathies. The neuromyopathies and peripheral neuropathies are most frequently encountered in patients harboring lung cancers.

## Encephalopathy

An example of one encephalopathy is progressive multifocal leukoencephalopathy, which is a relatively rare, acute, and widely disseminated demyelinating disorder that rapidly terminates in death. The symptoms include lethargy, stupor, dementia, and personality alterations. In contrast to the other neurogenic syndromes, this disease is usually seen in the lymphomas such as Hodgkin's disease, non-Hodgkin's lymphoma, and the myeloproliferative disorders. The etiology may be related to infection with a slow virus. The diagnosis is clinical but can also be made by brain biopsy. In the latter one sees diffuse involvement of the gray matter. A number of different clinical syndromes are associated, such as corticocerebellar degeneration, encephalomyelopathy, dementia, and memory loss. Other disease entities may mimic progressive multifocal leukoencephalopathy, such as meningeal carcinomatosis and CNS leukemia.

## Myelopathy

The myelopathy seen in patients with carcinoma is usually painless and of an acute or subacute onset, leading to sensory deficits with progressive development of paraplegia, anesthesia, and incontinence. It is usually fairly rare. One must rule out epidural metastatis or transverse myelitis or vascular infarction secondary to radiation therapy. It is most commonly associated with bronchogenic carcinoma but is also seen in ovarian and stomach cancer.

## Peripheral Neuropathy and Myopathy

The peripheral neuropathies are generally categorized by a group of disorders called *neuromyopathies*. Patients present with bilateral or unilateral proximal muscle wasting and weakness with a decrease or loss of the deep tendon reflexes. It may also be associated with a significant sensory component mimicking sciatica. Diagnosis can be made by EMG and measurement of the conduction velocity of affected peripheral nerves.

The myopathy usually presents as muscle fatigue and weakness. Metabolic abnormalities such as cachexia of malignancy may explain the weakness, and the possibility of a steroid myopathy should be considered in the differential diagnosis. However, primary muscle diseases do occur and in many cases affect the neuromuscular junction, such as in myasthenia gravis or the Eaton-Lambert syndrome. In myasthenia, which is usually associated with thymic tumors, characteristic features include weakness aggravated by exertion, diplopia, dysarthria, and dysphagia. Thymomas are usually present in 10% of these patients and should be treated surgically if at all possible. Another syndrome that is the reverse of myasthenia is the Eaton-Lambert syndrome where weakness is improved by exertion. It can be differentiated from true myasthenia by electromyographic studies where repetitive stimulation of action potentials results in an increase to normal levels. In myasthenia gravis repetitive stimulation of the action potentials shows a rapid decrease from normal to subnormal levels. The Eaton-Lambert syndrome is mainly seen in patients with carcinomas of the lung, including small-cell carcinoma and may precede the diagnosis of tumor by as much as one year. Effective treatment of the tumor is accompanied by remission of the syndrome.

Polymyositis and dermatomyositis may often be a coexisting accompaniment of malignancy. It may precede the diagnosis of tumor by as much as a year and the clinical effects are characteristically proximal muscle weakness, pain, and wasting of the muscles without reflex or sensory deficits. Both acute and chronic forms may occur. The diagnosis is made by the demonstration of very elevated levels of muscle enzymes such as CPK, aldolase, LDH, and SGOT, which generally return to normal with treatment. Dermatomyositis may accompany the polymyositis or may be an independent occurrence. The dermatomyositis associated with malignancy occurs in patients above the age of 50 years. Tumors associated with these syndromes include ovarian, breast, and uterine sites. Treatment of the primary tumor is helpful and in some cases high doses of Prednisone or immunosuppression with Cytoxan or Immuran is advised.

## OTHER CATEGORIES OF PARANEOPLASTIC SYNDROMES

We have already discussed pertubations in host physiology, endocrine –metabolic syndromes, and neurogenic–paraneoplastic syndromes. Other categories of paraneoplastic syndromes include alterations in hematopoiesis, altered coagulability of the blood, gastrointestinal cancer syndromes, and complications of cancer treatment. These are discussed briefly.

Alterations in hematopoiesis include the chronic anemias seen with cancers; sideroblastic anemias, as well as erythrocytosis due to indirect or direct effects of the tumor on the bone marrow, are seen. With regard to the former, elevated levels of erythropoietin have been described in patients harboring renal-cell carcinomas and hepatomas. Five cases of erythropoiesis secreting lung cancer have also been reported in the literature. The direct effects of the tumor on the bone marrow leading to either myelophthistic anemias or irritation of the bone marrow by tumor cells leading to a leucoerythroblastic blood picture have been described.

Altered coagulability may result from tumor effects on serum clotting factors or effects on platelet function or production. Changes in coagulability of the blood related to the production of prothrombin by the liver may be affected by direct involvement of the liver by tumor cells. Hypercoagulable states are often associated with pancreatic lung carcinomas, leading to migratory thrombophlebitis. Platelet function may be disturbed in patients with malignant disease and can be reflected as diffuse intravascular coagulation (DIC). This may be acute, such as in acute promyelocytic leukemia or chronic, such as in prostatic carcinomas involving the bone marrow.

Gastrointestinal cancer syndromes may be manifested as diarrhea, such as in the carcinoid syndrome or malabsorption, such as in direct invasion by lymphoma of the gastrointestinal tract. Certain drugs given at high doses, especially gut sterilization antibiotics, can also lead to malabsorption of food stuffs as well as chemotherapeutic agents. Hypergastrinemia due to pancreatic islet-cell tumors (Zollingen-Ellison syndrome) may cause multiple small-bowel ulceration. Diarrhea has also been seen in pancreatic islet-cell tumors as a result of secretion of vasoactive polypeptide. Protein-losing enteropathies may lead to hypoalbuminemia, as seen in patients with gastrointestinal neoplasms or lymphomas. Vincristine administration may lead to decreased peristalsis and then to constipation.

Finally, complications of cancer treatment may lead to a variety of paraneoplastic syndromes. Some of these have been discussed previously and include inappropriate ADH secretion secondary to Cytoxan and Vincristine administration as well as malabsorption secondary to gut sterilization antibiotics. The neurogenic complications described in association with Vincristine administration are usually reversible with a decrease in drug dosage or with cessation of drug administration. Other complications of cancer treatment include infectious complications due to depression of the immune system or white blood cells. Spermatogenesis has been found to be decreased in patients undergoing MOPP therapy for Hodgkin's and non-Hodgkin's lymphomas. Hyperkalemia may be seen in Burkitt cell tumors when sudden lysis may occur due to chemotherapy. The development of secondary malignancies in patients with Hodgkin's disease has often been associated with combined modality therapy with radiation and drugs.

In summary, various paraneoplastic syndromes have been recognized, many of which can be used as an index of tumor response or progression, therefore allowing one to capitalize on their presence. In general, one must be aware of the paraneoplastic syndromes, treat them rapidly and effectively, and be aware of the various syndromes that may be associated with the treatment itself.

## REFERENCES

1. McKendail AK: Remote effects of cancer on the nervous system. Rush Presbyt St Lukes Med Bull 11: 2, 1972.
2. Ross EJ: Endocrine and metabolic manifestation of cancer. Brit Med 1: 735, 1972.
3. Hall TC: Ed.: Paraneoplastic Syndromes. Proc NY Acad Sciences, 1974.
4. Holland J, Frei E, Eds.: Cancer Medicine. Lea & Febiger, Philadelphia, 1973.

5. Broder LE, Carter SK: Pancreatic islet cell carcinoma. I. Clinical features of 52 patients. Ann Intern Med 79: 101, 1973*a*.
6. Broder LE, Carter SK: Pancreatic islet cell carcinoma. II. Results of therapy with Streptozotocin in 52 patients. Ann Intern Med 79: 108, 1973*b*.
7. Williams RH, Ed.: Textbook of Endocrinology, 5th ed. Saunders, Philadelphia, 1974.
8. Broder LE, Weintraub BD, Rosen SW, Cohen MH, and Tesada F: Placental proteins and their subunits as tumor markers in prostatic carcinoma. Cancer 40: 211–216, 1977.
9. Rosen SW, Weintraub BD, Vaitukaitus JL, Sussman HH, Hershman JM, Muggia FM: Placental proteins and their subunits as tumor markers. Ann Int Med 82: 71–83, 1977.

# SURGICAL ONCOLOGY 1978: APPLICATIONS OF THE CONCEPT OF INTERDISCIPLINARY CANCER THERAPY

EVERETT V. SUGARBAKER, M.D.

## INTERDISCIPLINARY THERAPY: NEED DICTATED BY THE CHARACTERISTICS OF MALIGNANCY

Malignant tumors exhibit not only unrestrained local expansion but also invade locally and release viable cells that establish distant foci of neoplastic growth—termed *distant metastases* (Figure 1). These processes of invasion and metastasis, which hold fascination for the experimental oncologist, are the intrinsic characteristics of cancer that defeat the clinical oncologists and prove lethal to many patients (1).

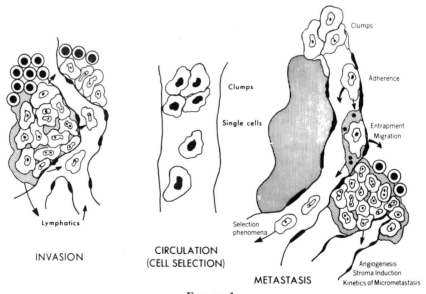

**FIGURE 1.**

Despite religious employment of the basic surgical principles of cancer management at the primary tumor site—which include wide radical resection, en bloc removal of regional lymph nodes, and use of various measures to prevent cancerous wound contamination—surgeons are still defeated by occult cancer cells undetectable by any known diagnostic method. The general logic of the interdisciplinary approach is, therefore, predicated on the intrinsic features of the disease process. These are: (1) the unrestrained primary tumor growth that continues to require aggressive surgical irradication and (2) the regional and distant subclinical extensions of these that require other therapy modalities.

The last several years have witnessed the simultaneous concatenation of: (1) experimental demonstration of the efficacy of adjuvant drug therapy, (2) the positive early results of adjuvant clinical trials, and (3) a broader understanding of the principles of the use of drug and/or radiotherapy as an adjuvant to surgical excision (2). The critical surgical question was whether the extent of this patient's disease rendered him operable. Although this question is an essential in surgical evaluation, the most significant question now is in regard to which combination of therapeutic modalities is needed not only to control the local and regional extensions of disease, but likewise to eradicate the occult systemic metastases. This blending of therapy modalities has been termed *interdisciplinary care*.

One of the most exciting current concepts in tumor biology is that there are therapeutically exploitable differences between primary tumors and micrometastases (Table 1). As is detailed in other presentations, micrometastases have a higher growth fraction, are better oxygenated, and constitute a lesser tumor or antigen burden than the

TABLE 1

*Therapeutic Exploitation of Differences Between Bulky Tumors and Micrometastases*

1. Tumor cell kinetics (i.e., higher growth fraction)
2. Vascularity (i.e., better oxygenated)
3. Immunologic (i.e., lesser tumor burden)
4. Other (i.e., thrombogenicity, angiogenicity, cytophysical)

primary tumor. These quantitative differences are being exploited in the design and application of interdisciplinary treatment programs.

There are several important categories in which successful interdisciplinary therapy is altering the actual practice of cancer surgery (Table 2). Each of these categories can be illustrated in the management of certain neoplastic diseases. In the future it is hoped that broader application of these modifications of the traditional cancer surgical approach will be found and proven effective.

## TABLE 2
### *Interdisciplinary Cancer Surgery*

1. Less ablative surgery may be possible when surgery is done for subclinical disease.

2. Need for the pathologic staging of regional nodes parallels therapeutic rationale.

3. Heroic procedures will have stronger rationale when effective adjuvants are available.

4. Cytoreductive surgery in selected patients with "localized disseminated disease."

## LESS ABLATIVE SURGERY MAY BE POSSIBLE WHEN SURGERY HAS BEEN DONE FOR SUBCLINICAL DISEASE

Limited excisions of soft-tissue sarcomas have been attended by local recurrence rates of 40–80% (3). This statistic fostered the application of radical amputation as a standard in soft-tissue sarcoma management in order to more greatly extend surgical margins and encompass the subclinical disease (3). However, the use of appropriate adjuvant radiotherapy has been shown to reduce recurrence rates to 14% in extremities sarcoma (4), a figure below that achievable even with radical amputation. Therefore, the standard of sarcoma management in the Division of Surgical Oncology at the University of Miami utilizes wide (but limb-preserving) excision and adjuvant radiotherapy wherever possible. Adjuvant chemotherapy for control of systemic metastasis is under study but not yet of demonstrated efficacy at this early time in follow-up.

Likewise, segmental resection of early breast carcinoma and adjuvant radiation therapy (5000 rads in 5 weeks) has been shown equally effective as traditional Halstead or modified radical mastectomy in the management of early breast cancer (5) and is being offered as an option in breast surgery in appropriate cases. The need for systemic adjuvant therapy is planned based on the pathologic analysis of axillary and/or internal mammary nodes removed by a simultaneous dissection.

## THE NEED FOR PATHOLOGIC STAGING OF REGIONAL LYMPH NODES PARALLELS A THERAPEUTIC RATIONALE FOR REMOVAL

In patients with malignant melanoma the prognosis is closely associated with the pathological presence or absence of metastatic regional nodes (6,7). If grossly positive nodes are present, survival is 20–25% at 5 years. If microscopically positive nodes only are present, survival is 45–60% at 5 years. However, if nodes are negative, survival is 75–85% at 5 years. These reported statistics would seem to substantiate the therapeutic application of elective regional node dissection in the treatment of malignant melanoma for microscopically present lymphatic disease. The prognosis when disease is caught in this stage is better than if nodes are grossly present. However, since only about 25–35% of all patients with clinically negative regional nodes have pathologically positive nodes and, since only a 20–30% increase in prognosis is achievable by operating on patients with microscopic nodes, the therapeutic benefit of this approach has been difficult to prove. In fact, early results of a World Health Organization randomized trial and a Mayo Clinic randomized trial have not yet shown statistical therapeutic benefit of elective node dissection for the management of malignant melanoma. However, if one is to select patients for adjuvant therapy and adequately stage the disease prior to adjuvant trials, the nodal status must be known. Therefore, in a protocol setting the staging rationale parallels the therapeutic rationale for node dissection. An identical argument can be made for removal of axillary lymph nodes in the management of carcinoma of the breast. At the University of Miami the possible efficacy of adjuvant *Corynebacterium parvum* is being explored in the management of malignant melanoma.

## Heroic Procedures Have a Stronger Rationale
## if Effective Adjuvant Therapy is Available

The disease-free interval of premenopausal women with carcinoma of the breast has been prolonged by the use of Cytoxan and Methotrexate and 5-Fluorouracil combined (CMF; *Bonadonna* regime). It is, therefore, possible to reconsider some of the interdictions of mastectomy generated by the clinical observations of the "surgery only" era of breast-cancer management. The Haagnsen criteria of inoperability (8), a valuable contribution in prechemotherapy management of breast cancer, must now be reexamined, for those women with local "C" or "D" lesions are usually doomed to local failure and death treated by palliative means. A radical resection to include the chest wall when required seems a rational consequence of successful chemotherapeutic management of distant micrometastases in these patients. In the era of successful adjuvant therapy, surgical technical expertise and prowess may well be rewarded by cure rather than by demise as was present in the prechemotherapeutic era.

## Cytoreductive Surgery in Selected Patients with
## Disseminated Disease May Be Indicated

Particularly in the management of massive malignant lymphomas, splenectomy and/or debulking procedures have significant rationale. By removal of infected extensive foci of disease, the chemotherapist's management is facilitated. It is to be emphasized that one must have an effective chemotherapeutic regime to make this type of surgical extirpation a reasonable alternative.

Clearly, longer observation intervals and additional data are required to solidify the efficacy of interdisciplinary therapy in many neoplastic processes. Ideal drug, surgical, and radiotherapeutic modality combinations need to be identified. Even if all patients were entered into protocols, the multiple stages of diseases and the myriad possibilities for adjuvant therapy would require many years of investigation. Therefore, it is important that as many patients as feasible be entered into appropriate protocolized management so that our questions in this regard can be answered in the foreseeable future.

# REFERENCES

1. Sugarbaker EV, Ketcham AS: Mechanism and prevention of metastasis of tumor dissemination in man—A surgeon's overview. Semin Oncol 4:19, 1977.
2. Sugarbaker EV, Ketcham AS, Zubrod GF: Interdisciplinary cancer therapy: Adjuvant therapy. Current Problems in Surgery, Ed. M. M. Ravitch. Year Book Medical Publishers, Chicago, 1977.
3. Cantin J, McNeer GP: The problem of local recurrence after treatment of soft tissue sarcoma. Ann Surg 168: 47, 1968.
4. Lindberg RD: The role of radiation therapy in the treatment of soft-tissue sarcoma in adults. Seventh National Cancer Conference Proceedings, 1973.
5. Harris JR, Levene MB, Hellman S, Loeber E: Definitive radiation for stage I & II carcinoma of the breast. Proc. ASCO 19: 314, 1978.
6. Sugarbaker EV, McBride CM: Melanoma of the trunk: The results of surgical excision and anatomic guidelines for predicting nodal metastasis. Surgery 80: 22, 1976.
7. Sugarbaker EV, McBride CM: Regional disease control and survival after isolation perfusion for invasive Stage I melanoma of the extremities (1958–1969). Cancer 37: 188, 1976.
8. Haagenson CD, Stout AP: Carcinoma of the breast: Criteria of operability. Ann Surg 118: 850, 1943.

# FUNDAMENTALS OF RADIATION THERAPY

KOMANDURI K. N. CHARYULU, M.D.

Ionizing radiations in the form of "X" and "gamma" rays (x-rays and γ-rays) or charged particles (electrons, protons, neutrons, and π-mesons), are employed in treating cancers. The incident radiations produce ions carrying positive or negative charges in the tissue upon interaction. As a result, highly reactive radicals are produced. These events in turn produce damage to the basic constituents of cell such as DNA, mitochondria, lysosomes, and cell membranes. The cell usually dies instantaneously, if the lethal damage is profound, or the subclinical damage associated with radiation could manifest in the subsequent generations of dividing cells and prove lethal to them.

Irradiation usually has differential effects on normal and malignant cells. The radiations act somewhat as a selective destructive tool against cancer cells, and not as a cautery of a block of tumor tissue that often has normal host tissues in addition. The success of radiation therapy at a cellular level depends on: (1) the differential radiosensitivity of malignant and normal cells, (2) the differential rates of division between the two types of cell population, and (3) the greater ability of normal cells to repair injury compared to cancer cells. The selective effect of radiation on cancers is determined by the usually higher rate of division of cancer cells with an associated greater degree of radiosensitivity as well as the incompetence of such cells to repair the damage. The irradiation of tissue thus produces death of cancer cells *in situ*. The host tissues are usually spared to a certain extent with the usual clinical doses that are commonly employed in the treatment of malignant conditions. Koller's early work in the 1950s reflects the role of host factors operating in conjunction with the ionizing radiation in eradicating malignant cells when the cancers are irradiated.

The two basic methods of delivering radiation for the treatment of cancer are: (1) External radiation therapy using (a) x-ray machines with or without electrons or (b) isotope machines and (2) internal radiation therapy as in (a) intracavitary therapy with applicators, or (b) interstitial radiation with radioactive seeds implanted in tissues.

## EXTERNAL RADIATION THERAPY

### X-ray

The x-rays commonly employed are in the range of 70,000 V (70 kV) to 40 million V (40 MV). In general, the higher the energy, the greater the penetration of x-rays. The low-kilovolt machines are used for treatment of skin and superficial cancer, while the deep-seated tumors such as in the trunk, are treated with the higher-energy machines. The x-rays can be classified into the following groups:

1. Superficial x-ray therapy, at 70,000–140,000 V (70–140 kV).
2. Deep x-ray therapy (orthovoltage), at 180,000–280,000 V (180–280 kV).
3. Supervoltage and megavoltage x-ray therapy, at $1 \times 10^6$ to $40 \times 10^6$ V (1000–40,000 kV). X-rays in this range have the advantages that skin reactions are spared and the doses to bone are less—unlike deep x-rays. Some of the supervoltage therapy units, while generating x-rays, also provide the high energy electrons for effective therapy of malignant lesions (21).

The machines generating the supervoltage or the megavoltage x-rays or electrons are known as linear accelerators and betatrons.

### Isotope Machines—$Co^{60}$ Teletherapy

The most common isotope employed is $Co^{60}$. The energy of γ-rays (same as x-rays) given by the decaying radioactive isotope is $1.2 \times 10^6$ V or 1.2 MV. The γ-radiation of a $Co^{60}$ teletherapy machine falls within the range of supervoltage x-ray therapy. The radiations given off by radioactive isotopes are usually the so-called γ-rays, although there is no difference between γ-rays and x-rays in respect to their action on tissues.

# INTERNAL RADIATION THERAPY

## Intracavitary Applications

The most important use of intracavitary radiation is in the management of cancers of the cervix (9), endometrium, and vagina. Less often, intracavitary radiation is used to treat cancers of the maxillary sinus and nasopharynx. Radioactive sources are often placed in applicators inserted under anesthesia.

## Interstitial Implants

The aim of the internal radiation therapy in this as well as intracavitary application is to concentrate the higher contribution of radiation dose to the site of origin of cancer where a bulk of tumor cells are present. In the interstitial implants, radioactive sources are implanted directly into the cancer such as in the tongue, oropharynx, tonsil, floor of the mouth, and other superficial areas easily accessible for such implants. The radioisotopes most frequently used are Ra, Rn seeds, $Au^{198}$ grains, and $I^{125}$ seeds.

## Systemic Therapy of Isotopes

Radioactive fluids such as radioactive phosphorus or radioactive $I^{131}$ are sometimes used by injection or by drink to treat the patients with polycythemia vera or carcinoma of the thyroid, respectively. Follicular carcinoma of the thyroid is often treated by $I^{131}$ solution given intraorally.

Rarely are radioactive fluids injected into the peritoneal or pleural cavities to eradicate pea-sized implants for cancerous tissue and to minimize the possibility of effusions into these serosal cavities. The isotopes used for this type of application are colloidal solutions of $Au^{198}$ or $P^{32}$.

## Units of Radiation Therapy

The roentgen is the unit for describing the amount of radiation given to a patient either as individual fraction or a number of fractions put together. However, this unit has limitations in terms of requiring measurement in an indirect manner, as "roentgen" only denotes exposure and not the dose absorbed by the tissue. Hence, another unit known as the "rad" was described that related directly with the absorption of dose in tissues. This abbreviation implies "radiation-absorbed dose." This unit stands for 100 ergs absorbed in 1 gram of tissue. One rad is not equal to one roentgen, as their relationship depends on the energy of the beam and the texture of the tissue radiated.

The dose of radiation is not given as a single dose as in many cases, but is administered as a number of fractions given over a certain period of time. It is customary to give five treatments per week over a period of several weeks. The usual doses commonly given in the curative range are 6000–6600 rads in 6–6½ weeks, the daily fraction being 200 rads per day. However, where the volume irradiated is large, the fraction given each day is dropped to 180 rads or less, depending on the size of the volume. Palliative doses are usually given in the range of up to 3000–4000 rads in 3–4 weeks. Although these doses in relation to overall time were originally based on empiricism, they are now subjected to both theoretical and experimental analysis (2,6,7,10). The statement of total dose is meaningless without knowledge of the overall treatment time and the number of fractions in which the dose is given. Although the tissues tolerate a dose of up to 6000–6600 rads in any one course, retreatment is possible depending on the treatment-free interval.

Tissue exhibiting sensitivity to irradiation are, in decreasing order: lymphoid, bone marrow, spermatic and ovarian epithelium, intestinal epithelium, optic lens, oropharyngeal epithelium, prostate, urinary bladder and urethral epithelium, renal epithelium, and muscular and neuronal tissue. The radiosensitivity is governed additionally by the degree of differentiation of tumor cells, stage of cell division, presence of oxygen around the cells, and temperature of the environment of the cells. Poorly differentiated tumors and anaplastic tumors have higher radiosensitivity than do well-differentiated neoplasms. Cells in mytosis are most radiosensitive compared to the stage immediately thereafter.

Cells with an abundant supply of oxygen are three times more radiosensitive than those that are anoxic (1). The later concept provides the rationale for administering radiation therapy in multiple fractions as the tumor cells are likely to be reoxygenated between fractions (5).

### Law of Bergonie and Tribondeau

This law states that x-radiations are most effective on those cells that: (1) have a greater reproductive activity, (2) have a longer dividing future ahead, and (3) whose morphology and function are least fixed. The more differentiated the tumor is, the smaller the fraction of actively proliferating tumor cells; the converse is true for anaplastic neoplasms.

Clinical radiosensitivity also depends on the size of the tumor and absence or presence of infection. The larger the size of the tumor, the greater the dose required to eradicate it (3,4,17,18). If there is simultaneous infection, the less effective is a given dose of radiation. Also, any anemic state of the patient contributes to decrease in radiosensitivity of tumor cells (8). In the context of the foregoing discussion is the observation that tumours regressing totally by the end of a curative course of radiotherapy have a better chance of permanent eradication (20).

The differential destructive effects on neoplastic tissues and normal tissues is related by what is known as "therapeutic ratio" (12). A given regimen of therapy is stated to have a high therapeutic ratio when the lethal effect on neoplastic tissue is highest, while the effect on normal tissue is the lowest. A high therapeutic ratio in practice is often accomplished by arranging multiple ports of radiation often targeting onto the tumor in several directions. Thus the dose of radiation to the entry port is distributed over several ports, while the beams traverse the tumor through all these ports. Intricate planning often minimizes the damage to the normal tissues, while enhancing the tumor lethal effect. Computers are essential tools in the efficient planning of a given treatment course.

### Preoperative and Postoperative Radiotherapy

The postoperative radiotherapy is given to eradicate clinical disease left at the time of surgical excision. If no postoperative radiotherapy is given, such cells often manifest as local recurrences. The postoperative radiation therapy simply bathes the tissues in the surgical field and is aimed at eradicating the remaining cells.

Radiation can be employed alone where the tumors are in an early stage. In such cases both the primary and lymph-node drainage areas are usually treated simultaneously to eradicate the primary tumor as well as the subclinical disease in the lymph nodes. However, where the tumors are large, combined modalities are more effective in eradicating the tumor and keeping the patients under control for long periods of time.

The preoperative radiation therapy is aimed at: (1) shrinking the tumor and rendering the tumor operable, (2) destroying the cells in the periphery that are often responsible for the spread of metastases at the time of dissection, (3) preventing implantation of cells at the primary site, and (4) minimizing the amount of dissemination during the surgical procedures (13,14,15,16). Beneficial results have been reported following preoperative radiotherapy in carcinoma of endometrium and supraglottic larynx (11,19).

There are side effects to the course of radiation therapy as for any other therapeutic modality. These side effects have to be weighed against the risk of failure to control the disease. They are usually seen with the higher doses that are necessary to eradicate the disease. Many of these radiation-induced reactions such as moist desquamation of the skin, mucositis of oral cavity, rectum, or vagina, and nausea, vomiting, and diarrhea usually subside after the completion of therapy. However, where higher doses of radiation must be given, a few long-term late complications are inevitable.

The use of treatment simulators, computers, and other treatments in the modern practice enables the radiation therapist to treat the malignancies while minimizing the probability of complications.

Curative radiation alone is employed in head and neck cancer, carcinoma of the larynx, Hodgkin's disease, seminomas of the testes, skin cancers, and carcinoma of the cervix.

Surgery and radiation therapy together have been employed in the management of head and neck cancers, testicular neoplasm, ovarian neoplasms, and carcinoma of the endometrium, along with certain abdominal malignancies.

Chemotherapy and irradiation are together employed in the management of patients with lymphomas, acute lymphatic leukemia, Ewing's sarcoma, and some brain, head, and neck neoplasms. Certain chemicals are used to enhance the radiosensitivity of tumor cells. These are Actinomycin-D and Hydroxyuria. Other chemotherapeutic regimens are being tried in conjunction with radiation therapy in many solid tumors.

Surgery, radiation therapy, and chemotherapy are together employed in the treatment of patients with Wilms's tumor, some testicular carcinomas, and soft-tissue sarcomas. Multiple modality therapies are certainly indicated in an aggressive approach against the management of malignant diseases.

Radiation therapy is an effective palliative agent in symptoms such as mediastinal compression, spinal-cord compression pain associated with bone metastases, and symptomatology associated with bronchogenic carcinoma. Dramatic relief can sometimes be obtained in patients suffering from mediastinal or spinal-cord compression, especially when these syndromes are associated with rapidly proliferating tumor tissues.

Radiation therapy is certainly one of the most important tools in the armamentarium against cancer having a useful role in the management of cancer.

## REFERENCES

1. Churchill-Davidson I, Sanger C, Thomlinson RH: Oxygenation in radiotherapy. II. Clinical application. Brit J Radiol 30: 406, 1957.
2. Du Sault LA: The influence of the time factor on the dose response curve. Am J Roentgenol, Rad Ther, Nucl Med 87: 567, 1962.
3. Elkind MM: Cellular aspects of tumor therapy. Radiology 74: 529, 1960.
4. Elkind MM, Sutton H: Radiation response of mammalian cells grown in culture. Radiat Res 13: 556, 1960.
5. Elkind MM: Reoxygenation and its potential in radiotherapy. In Brookhaven National Laboratory: Proceedings of Conference on Time and Dose Relationships in Radiation Biology as Applied in Radiotherapy, Carmel, California, 1969, BNL50203 (C-57), p. 318.
6. Ellis F: The relationship of biological effect to dose in time-fractionation factors in radiotherapy. In Current Topics in Radiation Research. Ed. M. Ebert and A. Howard. Wiley, New York, 1968, Vol. 4, p. 357.

7. Ellis F: Nominal standard dose and ret. Brit J Radiol 84: 101, 1971.

8. Evans JC, Bergsjo P: The influence of anemia on results of radiotherapy in carcinoma of the cervix. Radiology 84:709, 1965.

9. Fletcher GH: Cancer of uterine cervix. Am J Roentgenol, Rad Ther, Nucl Med 111: 225, 1971.

10. Fowler JF: Experimental animal results relating to time in dose relationships in radiotherapy and the "ret" concept. Brit J Radiol 44: 81, 1971.

11. Hendrickson FR, Liebner E: Results of pre-operative radiotherapy for supraglottic larynx cancer. Ann Otol 77:222, 1968.

12. Hewitt HB: Fundamental aspects of the radiotherapy of cancer. Sci Basis Med Ann Rev, 305, 1962.

13. Hoye RCM, Smith PR: Effectiveness of small amount of preoperative irradiation in preventing the growth of tumor cells disseminated at surgery. Cancer 14: 284, 1961.

14. Perez CA, Olson J: Preoperative versus postoperative irradiation: comparison in experimental animal tumor system. Am J Roentgenol, Rad Ther, Nucl Med 108: 396, 1970.

15. Perez CA, Powers WE: Studies on the optimal dose of preoperative irradiation and time for surgery in the cure of a mouse lymphosarcoma. Radiology 89: 116, 1967.

16. Powers WE, Palmer LA: Biologic basis of preoperative radiation treatment. Am J Roentgenol, Rad Ther, Nucl Med 102: 176, 1968.

17. Puck TT, Marcus PI: Actions of x-rays on mammalian cells. J Exp Med 103:653, 1956.

18. Puck TT, Morkovon D, Marcus PI, Cieciura SJ: Action of x-rays on mammalian cells. II. Survival curves of cells from normal tissues. J Exp Med 106: 485, 1957.

19. Sudarsanam A, Charyulu K, Hintz B, Averette H, Belinson J: Adjuvant preoperative external irradiation with or without intracavitary radium in the management of endometrial carcinoma. In Adjuvant Therapy of Cancer. Ed. S. E. Salmon and S. E. Jones. North Holland Publishing Co., Amsterdam, Oxford, New York, 335, 1977.

20. Suit H, Lindberg R, Fletcher GH: Prognostic significance of extent of tumor regression at completion of radiation therapy. Radiology 84: 1100, 1965.

21. Tapley NV, Fletcher GH: Patterns of use of 6-18 MeV electron beam radiation therapy. Am J Roentgenol, Rad Ther, Nucl Med 99: 924, 1967.

# FUNDAMENTAL AND CLINICAL ASPECTS OF CANCER CHEMOTHERAPY

HOWARD E. LESSNER, M.D.

## BACKGROUND

The modern era of cancer chemotherapy began in the 1940s with the introduction of the folic acid antagonists and gathered force in the mid-1950s with the continuing introduction of the alkylating agents and the development of the National Cancer Chemotherapy Program. The past 20 years have seen the development of a new specialty, cancer chemotherapy, usually administered by a trained medical oncologist. In part, the rapid emergence of this newly recognized subspecialty stems from recognition of the inability of both the surgeon and the radiotherapist to cure all cancer patients, even when the diagnosis is made relatively early, and in part is due to the increasing therapeutic effectiveness of chemotherapeutic agents and combinations thereof. Gradually there has evolved a fund of knowledge, both clinical and experimental, on which the present principles of cancer therapy are dependent. The most important of these principles may be briefly summarized as follows:

1. Despite the many advances in chemotherapeutic management, surgery and radiotherapy remain the "curative" modalities of cancer therapy in the overwhelming majority of potentially curable patients.
2. The growth of most tumors is related more to the accumulation of long-lived cells than to either rapid cellular proliferation in the tumor or to a large growth fraction (i.e., % of total cells in active cellular replication phase) (1). Those tumors with a rela-

56

tively high growth fraction (e.g., Burkitt's lymphoma, chorio-carcinoma, acute leukemias) are generally most susceptible to chemotherapeutic treatment, whereas tumors with relatively low growth fractions and cellular kinetics similar to normal tissues are correspondingly more difficult to treat.

3. The lethality of tumors is generally, although not always, related to the total tumor mass, and it has been estimated that approximately $10^{12}$ tumor cells approaches a lethal level in man (2). The therapeutic aims of cancer treatment are directed at reducing this total tumor load. In general, chemotherapeutic reduction of total tumor mass to 50% of the original value will result in prolongation of life in the recipient regardless of the type of tumor (3).

4. Tumor-cell destruction by chemotherapy is a logarithmic function similar to that of bacterial destruction by appropriate antibiotics (3). Generally, drugs presently available are capable of 2–3 logs of cell kill (i.e., $10^{11}$ reduced to $10^8$ cells). Since a mass containing $10^9$ cells is at the lower limit of clinical detectability (i.e., 1 cm in diameter), it is clear that patients with less than $10^9$ cells in a single tumor mass will have clinically undetectable disease, even though substantial numbers of tumor cells are present. Thus the concept of microfoci of tumor cells (micrometastatic disease) is universally accepted with the accompanying axiom that most metastatic disease occurs sometime before the primary tumor is detected.

5. Many investigators have attempted to quantitate the doubling time of tumor masses, and most of these studies deal with timed measurements of discernible masses with extrapolation back to the presumed single cancer cell. These observations have indicated that in most cases the larger the tumor mass becomes, the slower the doubling time. This phenomenon may be related to external pressures, poor vascularity, or inhibition of tumor-cell replication by adjacent tumor cells. Some have suggested, on the basis of such calculations, that there may be a period of 10–15 years from the time that the original mutation occurs and the primordial cell becomes cancerous, until it becomes clinically evident. It is thus clear why even prompt removal of primary tumors is sometimes ineffective in curing cancer.

These general principles of cancer-cell kinetics, lethality, and growth characteristics have changed significantly our understandings and approaches to the treatment of cancer. It is apparent that hope for cure or long-term palliation in many situations must reside in therapeutic attacks designed to counteract the above-mentioned data. Such strategies would include the following:

1. The institution of systemic treatment as early as possible in those localized cancers surgically removable but statistically reported to have a high rate of recurrence. Such an approach is designed to eradicate micrometastatic disease prior to its clinical reappearance, and many such studies have recently been reported in diseases such as breast carcinoma (4,5), colon carcinoma (6), osteosarcoma (7,8), and so on. The early results in breast cancer and osteosarcomas seem encouraging, at least in certain subcategories of these diseases, but much more data will be necessary to properly evaluate this approach.
2. Use of more intensive or more prolonged chemotherapy to discourage the emergence of resistent clones of cancer cells. This might include high doses of a single drug such as recent studies involving enormous doses of Methotrexate with Citrovorum Rescue, which have been quite encouraging in certain types of carcinomas and sarcomas (8). Combinations of drugs that are not mutually additive toxicologically but have cumulative killing effect on cancer cells are also used extensively by skilled chemotherapists (9,10). Such combinations, which have almost achieved the status of "standard therapy," abound in the literature and generally are more advantangeous to the patients in terms of improved response rates than single drug programs.

Increasing the period of chemotherapy administration is an attempt to progressively lower the tumor-cell burden to a point where the body's natural defense mechanisms might be capable of eradicating the remaining tumor cells. Such approaches in acute leukemias (11) and lymphoma (12), utilizing 6–18 months of therapy are relatively standard. Intensive chemotherapy is continued for many months beyond clinical remission. A similar technique is being used with breast cancer and with many of the childhood tumors.

3. Finally, the use of varying combinations of surgery, chemotherapy, and radiation therapy in an attempt to obviate all macroscopic as well as microscopic disease is receiving intensive investigation; this is the so-called multimodal approach to treatment. It will be some time, perhaps years, before the true clinical value of such efforts becomes statistically assessable.

4. The concept of sanctuary sites has developed from the clinical observations of occurrence of meningeal leukemia and lymphomas in patients who are otherwise in complete remission (13). Such sites are presumed to be locations wherein tumor cells are protected from lethal doses of chemotherapy because of a perfusion barrier (e.g., the CNA blood–brain barrier system). The usual approach to this problem involves either the use of central nervous system intrathecal therapy with drugs such as Methotrexate or CNS radiation therapy in those disease states wherein this is a high-risk problem (e.g., acute leukemias, small-cell carcinoma of lung).

5. Cure of cancer is probably dependent on eradicating every residual cancer cell in the body, either through surgery, radiation, chemotherapy or the body's own immunological defense system. It is believed that if the tumor burden is lowered sufficiently (ca. $10^3$ cells), then the host's immunodefense system might be able to destroy the remaining cells. Major immunodefense treatment programs have been aimed at boosting immunologic resistence in the host using both nonspecific and/or specific immunosimulation such as BCG and/or allogenic tumor cells. Such efforts have been tried in a number of human cancers, most commonly in melanomas (14) and leukemias (15), but it is too early as yet for a clear-cut assessment of effectiveness.

## CANCER CHEMOTHERAPY

Keeping in mind the above comments, it is appropriate at this time to generally review the major classes of available agents, although a complete summary of the present chemotherapeutic approaches to human cancer is beyond the scope of this chapter. For maximum clarity it is easiest to divide the chemotherapeutic agents into a variety of types depending on chemical natures and their mechanisms of action:

### Alkylating Agents (16)

These compounds, examples of which are Mustargen, Cytoxan, Alkeran, Leukeran, and Myleran, are called "alkylating" agents because of their ability to attach short alkyl chains to nucleophilic sites on biologic materials. The target biologic materials are macromolecules such as DNA and RNA, and the effect of attachment to several base sites in these molecules is disruption of the chains. Since these compounds attack preformed macromolecules, they are categorized as *cell cycle nonspecific agents*.

In general, these agents are all myelotoxic and the rapidity of response, and toxicity is more dependent on the method of administration of the drug than the specific drug itself. Intravenous drug administration generally depresses the counts in 7–14 days, with the major therapeutic effects being seen in 2–3 weeks. Oral administration of these compounds given on a chronic administration basis cause more delayed myelosuppression, usually taking 3–6 weeks to reach a nadir, with a correspondingly slower response. There are generally only minor differences in the therapeutic effectiveness of these agents, and resistance to adequate doses of one alkylating agent almost always implies resistance to the others.

For the sake of brevity the various drugs are listed in Table 1 with their method of administration and the types and degrees of toxicity

**TABLE 1**

*Toxicity of the Major Alkylating Agents*

| DRUG | ADMINIS-TRATION | N & V | MYELO-TOXICITY | LOCAL VESICANT | ALOPECIA | HEMOR-RHAGIC CYSTITIS | PULMO-NARY FIBROSIS |
|---|---|---|---|---|---|---|---|
| Mustargen | IV | ++++ | ++++ | ++++ | ō | ō | ō |
| Cytoxan | IV | +++ | ++++ | ō | +++ | ++ | + |
|  | PO |  | +++ | − | ++ | ++ | + |
| Leukeran | PO | + | +++ | − | ō | ō | ō |
| Alkeran | PO | + | +++ | − | ō | ō | ō |
| Myleran | PO | + | ++++ | − | ō | ō | ++ |

that might be expected. Of interest is the relatively specific toxic effect of alopecia and the hemorrhagic cystitis seen with Cytoxan and the occasional pulmonary fibrosis seen in patients given Myleran and more rarely, Cytoxan.

The aklylating agents have been used in all types of human malignancy, and almost all chemotherapeutically treatable tumors respond in some measure to these agents. They have been found to be most useful in: (1) lymphoproliferative disorders, (2) myeloproliferative disorders, (3) adenocarcinoma of the breast, (4) adenocarcinoma of the ovaries, and (5) carcinoma of the lung.

## Antimetabolites (17–20)

Methotrexate, 6-Mercaptopurine, Ara-C, 5-Fluorouracil (5-FU), and 6-Thioguanine are compounds that interfere with the metabolic pathways in cellular replication (notably, production of DNA and RNA). These compounds are thus termed *cell cycle specific*, the agents evidencing their major activity during the S (synthesis) phase of the cell cycle. Since these compounds are most active during cellular replication, they are of greatest value in high growth rate tumors having the largest proportions of cells in active replication phases such as the acute leukemias and choriocarcinoma. As there are major differences in action, specificity, and toxicity within this group of compounds it is appropriate to discuss these agents individually.

*Methotrexate (17)*   This agent inhibits the conversion of folic acid to active cofactor by irreversibly binding dihydrofolate reductase. This in turn prevents single carbon transfers necessary in the formation of pyrimidine and purine molecules and in the formation of certain proteins. This drug is unique in that it is metabolized to a minimal degree in the body and is excreted almost completely through the kidneys by glomerular filtration and tubular transport mechanisms. Thus, since the activity of the compound is directly proportional to its serum half-life, any impairment of renal function markedly prolongs the levels of circulating Methotrexate, increasing toxicity accordingly. Resistance to the compound occurs through two major mechanisms, an increase in cellular content of the target enzyme dihydrofolate reductase and a decrease in membrane permeability to Methotrexate. The toxicity of the drug is related directly to the duration of exposure and to the dose level.

Methotrexate and its congeners has been utilized longer than any other chemotherapeutic agents in the treatment of human malignancy, but its ultimate role is still not settled. Whereas it was most frequently utilized in acute leukemias of children, more recent developments utilizing different drug schedules and dosages have served to exemplify the importance of such manipulations in determining the maximum effectiveness of chemotherapeutic agents.

Doses and schedules vary widely from 2–5 mg/d to 20–30 g given intermittently with Leucovorin Rescue. Readers may find recommended schedules in sections of this volume dealing with specific disease entities. Very high doses ($\leq$ 30 g/d) with "rescue" by Citrovorum Factor has recently received much attention in the treatment of sarcomas, head and neck tumors, and leukemias (8,21).

The major toxic reactions to Methotrexate include bone-marrow depression, mucositis, diarrhea, alopecia, and occasionally a maculopapular rash. Hepatic fibrosis has been seen with chronic administration and high doses may produce irreversible renal damage.

*Antipurines* These agents, such as 6-Mercaptopurine (6-MP) and 6-Thioguanine (6-TG), act as negative feedback inhibitors of purine synthesis. 6-Thioguanine incorporates additionally into the DNA purine base. Mechanisms of resistance to these drugs in humans are uncertain, though they may be related to failure to convert the drugs to the ribonucleotides. 6-Mercaptopurine is oxidized by Xanthine Oxidase and thus the concomitant use of Allopurinol, an inhibitor of xanthine oxidase, is an indication for decreasing the dose of 6-MP significantly. 6-Thioguanine, on the other hand, is metabolized to a methylated derivative and thus is not potentiated by Allopurinol. Both 6-MP and 6-TG are given orally and produce toxicity including bone-marrow depression, nausea, vomiting, macropapular skin eruptions, and occasionally centrolobular necrosis of the liver. The clinical usefulness of the antipurines is almost entirely limited to the acute leukemias.

*Pyrimidine Antagonists—5-Fluorouracil (5-FU) and Arabinosyl Cytosine (Ara-C)* 5-Fluorouracil inhibits thymidilate synthetase and also is incorporated into spurious DNA. This compound has been administered by various means, the most common being an intravenous intermittent loading schedule of 4–5 days of treatment. Recent studies indicate that such a dose schedule is probably better than a weekly one, although some dispute continues regarding this point. 5-Fluorouracil has also been used orally, but most investigators have now discarded this method of administration as being inferior to intravenous usage. In addition, a topical 5-FU ointment has been applied locally to basal-cell carcinomas and premalignant keratoses with good effect.

5-Fluorouracil produces bone-marrow depression, nausea, anorexia, mucositis, diarrhea, skin rash, and occasional cerebellar ataxia and alopecia. It has been used mainly in gastrointestinal tract malignancies, where it has been the mainstay of treatment despite the fact that the level of efficacy is only in the range of 15–20% responses. It has also been used with good effect in breast cancer, both alone and in combination, and has limited usefulness in gynecological malignancies and prostatic carcinoma.

Another pyrimidine antagonist is Arabinosyl Cytosine (Ara-C, Cytarabine), which is an analog of deoxycytidine. The mechanism of action of this compound is not clear, although it is probably incorporated into spurious RNA and DNA. The drug is inactivated by deamination and thereafter excreted into the urine in an inactive form. It may be given intravenously or subcutaneously and produces similar toxicity to 5-FU. The major usefulness of Arabinosyl Cytosine is in the adult acute leukemias in combination with other agents (20).

**The Alkaloids**

These compounds are extracted from plants, prime examples of which are Vinblastine and Vincristine (24,25). The mechanism of action of these compounds is not clearly understood, although they have been shown to inhibit the cell cycle at metaphase, and have toxic effects during the S phase and possibly during the $G_2$ resting phase. These compounds crystallize microtubular and spindle proteins, and this effect is thought to explain the dose-limiting neurotoxicity of Vincristine. Table 2 describes the method of administration and major toxic potentials of these two compounds. Neurotoxicity is characterized by loss of reflexes, digital parasthesias, circumoral dysthesia, autonomic dysfunction (constipation and abdominal pain), paresis, inappropriate ADH secretion, and occasional coma. It is interesting that Vinblastine is a much more severe bone-marrow suppressant than Vincristine but

## TABLE 2
### *Toxicity of the Plant Alkaloids*

| DRUG | ADMINIS- TRATION | LOCAL VESICANT | MARROW SUPP. | NEUROTOXIC | ALOPECIA |
|---|---|---|---|---|---|
| Vinblastine | IV | ++++ | +++ | ± | ± |
| Vincristine | IV | ++++ | ± | ++++ | +++ |

Neurotoxicity: loss of reflexes, parasthesias, autonomic dysfunction (constipation and abdominal pain), paresis, inappropriate ADH secretion, and coma.

that Vincristine is much more difficult to administer because of its severe neurotoxic potential.

The major usefulness of these compounds is for the lymphoproliferative disorders. Vincristine is most used in acute lymphocytic leukemia, lymphocytic lymphomas, and Hodgkin's disease, while Velban is used almost exclusively for Hodgkin's disease because of its relatively specific effectiveness. Vincristine, because of its unique lack of marrow-toxic effect, is used extensively in combination drug programs, most effectively in breast and testicular tumors, choriocarcinomas, and childhood tumors.

### The Antitumor Antibiotics

These are microbial products that have the capacity to inhibit tumor cellular growth. Most of these compounds are derived from varieties of streptomycetes strains. They function at the molecular level, generally by intercalating between strands of nucleic acids, inhibiting synthesis and causing scission of macromolecular strands. Each antibiotic has its own particular spectrum of activity, and there are significant differences in toxicologic potential. Table 3 summarizes the major drugs used in clinical practice, and Table 4 describes some of the more common toxicologic potentials of these highly toxic compounds. It is of interest that Bleomycin has very little bone-marrow toxicity but does produce pulmonary fibrosis, skin rashes, fever, and mucositis quite frequently. Daunomycin and Adriamycin are very similar; both are severe vesicants and produce bone-marrow depression, alopecia, fever, nausea, vomiting, mucositis, and most specifically, cardiomyopathy and cardiac arrhythmias (24,25). The cardiac arrhythmic effect

**TABLE 3**

*Antitumor Antibiotics—Mechanism of Action*

| DRUG | MECHANISM OF ACTION | COMMENTS |
|------|--------------------|---------| 
| Actinomycin-D (10) | Binds to DNA, inhibits DNA-dependent RNA polymerase | |
| Adriamycin (11) | Intercalates between strands of DNA preventing duplication | Significantly excreted in bile—lower dose if hepatic function impaired |
| Daunomycin (12) | " | No dose variation needed with hepatic disease |
| Bleomycin (13) | Reacts with DNA causing strand scission | Concentrated in skin and lung, inactivated by all other organs |

of Daunomycin and Adriamycin is not dose related and may occur after even the first administration of the drugs (26). However, the cardiomyopathy of these drugs is dose related and is the result of myofibrillar degeneration caused by these compounds. The cumulative toxicity is nonreversible and may result in refractory congestive heart failure. The usefulness of these compounds is summarized in Table 5. Of most interest is the effectiveness of Adriamycin in the lymphomas, mesenchymal tumors, breast carcinoma, ovarian cancer, and certain types of lung cancers (24,27). Daunomycin is specifically used in the treatment of acute myelocytic and myelomonocytic leukemia (25).

**TABLE 4**

*Toxicity of the Antitumor Antibiotics*

| DRUG | ADMINIS-TRATION | MARROW SUPP. | LOCAL VESICANT | ALOPECIA | SKIN RASH | N & V | MU-COSI-TIS | OTHER |
|------|-----------------|--------------|----------------|----------|-----------|-------|-------------|-------|
| Actinomycin-D | IV | + + + + | + + + | + + + | + + | + + | + + + | |
| Daunomycin | IV | + + + + | + + + + | + + + + | + + + | + + | + + + | (1) |
| Adriamycin | IV | + + + + | + + + + | + + + + | + + + | + + | + + + | (1) |
| Bleomycin | IV & IM | + | − | + + | + + + | + | + + + | (2) |

*(1)*Cardiac arrhythmias and cardiomyopathy.
*(2)*Pulmonary interstitial fibrosis.

**TABLE 5**

*Major Clinical Uses of the Antitumor Antibiotics*

| AGENT | DISORDER |
|---|---|
| Actinomycin-D | Choriocarcinoma |
| | Testicular tumors—except seminomas, usually in combination |
| | Wilms's tumor |
| | Embryonal rhabdomyosarcoma |
| Daunomycin | Acute myelocytic leukemia |
| | Acute monocytic leukemia |
| Adriamycin | Lymphomas |
| | Breast carcinoma |
| | Lung carcinoma (in combination) |
| | Sarcomas (in combination) |
| | Testicular tumors |
| | Ovarian carcinoma |
| Bleomycin | Squamous-cell carcinomas |
| | Lymphomas |
| | Testicular tumors |

Bleomycin, following rather overenthusiastic initial reports, has now been found to be of most usefulness in lymphomas and in testicular carcinomas generally when used as part of a combination drug program.

**The Nitrosoureas**

Examples of these are BCNU, CCNU, Methyl-CCNU, and Streptozotocin. These compounds probably act as alkylating agents, although their exact mechanism of action is still somewhat obscure. Some of these drugs have just been released for general medical usage, although Methyl-CCNU and Streptozotocin are still restricted to experimental treatment programs. These agents are lipid soluble and nonionizable and as such effectively penetrate the blood–brain barrier. They are often used in combination programs since major bone-marrow toxicity is delayed 4–6 weeks and does not overlap bone-marrow toxicity from most other classes of compounds. Streptozotocin and BCNU are given intravenously, and Methyl-CCNU and CCNU are given orally. Most of these compounds, as noted above, are severely marrow-toxic, taking 4–6 weeks to reach count nadirs. They all may cause some nausea and vomiting, Streptozotocin producing this most severely. Streptozotocin is not myelotoxic but does produce significant renal toxicity. Those agents given intravenously are local vesicants and must be handled with care.

The nitrosoureas are effective in Hodgkin's disease and histiocytic lymphomas, generally being used in combination programs (28). An approximately 30–35% response rate has been found for BCNU in CNS tumors, and this is probably the most effective single chemotherapeutic agent we have for these tumors. These agents have also been found to be of value in multiple myeloma, certain lung cancer, and gastrointestinal-tract malignancies. Streptozotocin is the most effective agent known for the treatment of pancreatic islet-cell carcinomas and carcinoids (29).

## Miscellaneous Agents

An example is dimethyl triazeno imidazole carboxamide (DTIC) (30). This drug has recently become clinically available and probably functions as an alkylating agent, perhaps through degradation to an alkyl group. It is absorbed poorly from the gastrointestinal tract and is hence given intravenously. One of its major toxic effects is nausea and vomiting, but it also may produce bone-marrow depression. The major usefulness of DTIC is in malignant melanoma, where it is the agent of choice with approximately a 20–25% response rate. It has also been useful in Hodgkin's disease, especially in those patients resistant to more standard chemotherapy.

## Combination Therapy

It is beyond the scope of this review to discuss the many combinations and permutations of the above-mentioned compounds, which are presently in use in the chemotherapeutic armamentarium. Such combinations require expert surveillance and constant dose adjustments to prevent severe toxic reactions, and readers wishing a general review of the subject are directed to reference (9). Some examples of such programs are contained in portions of this book dealing with specific disease states.

## REFERENCES

1. Stell GG: Cytokinetics of neoplasia. *In* Cancer Medicine, Ed. J. F. Holland and E. Frei, Lea & Febiger, Philadelphia, 1973, p. 125.
2. DeVita V, Young RC, Canellos GP: Combination versus single agent chemotherapy. A review of the basis for selection of drug treatment of cancer. Cancer 35: 98, 1975.
3. Schabel FM: Concepts for systemic treatment of micrometastases. Cancer 35: 15, 1975.
4. Fisher B, Carbone P, Economou SG, et al: 1-Phenylalanine mustard (L-PAM) in the management of primary breast cancer, A report of early findings. NEJM 292: 117, 1975.
5. Bonadonna G, Brusamolino E, Valagussa P, Rossi A, Brugnatelli L, Brambilla C, DeLena M, Tancini G, Bajetta E, Musumeis R, Veronesi U: Combination chemotherapy as an adjuvant treatment in operable breast cancer. NEJM 294: 406, 1976.
6. Higgins GA, Dwight RW, Smith JV, Keehn RJ: Fluorouracil as an adjuvant to surgery in carcinoma of the colon. Arch Surg 102: 339, 1971.
7. Cortes EP, Holland JF, Wang JJ, Sinks LF, Blom J, Sinn H, Bank A, Glidewell O: Amputation and Adriamycin in primary osteogenic sarcoma. NEJM 291: 998, 1974.
8. Jaffe N, Traggis D: Toxicity of high dose Methotrexate (NSC-740) and citrovorum factor (NSC-3590) in osteogenic sarcoma. Cancer Chemother Rep Part 3, 6: 31, 1975.
9. DeVita VT, Schern PS: The use of drugs in combination for the treatment of cancer. New Surg J Med 288: 998, 1973.
10. Cooper R: Combination chemotherapy in hormonal resistant breast Ca. Proc Am Assoc Cancer Res 10: 15, 1969.
11. Frei E: Combination cancer therapy. Presidential address. Cancer Res 32: 2593, 1972.
12. DeVita V, Canellos G, Hubbard S, Chabner B, Young R: Chemotherapy of Hodgkin's disease (H.D.) with MOPP. A 10 year progress report. ASCO Abstracts C-131: 269, 1976.
13. Aur RJA, Simone J, Husto HO et al: Central nervous system therapy and combination chemotherapy of childhood lymphocytic leukemia. Blood 37:272, 1971.
14. Eilber FR, Morton DL, Holmes EC et al.: Adjuvant immunotherapy with BCG in treatment of regional lymphnode metastasis from malignant melanoma. NEJM 294: 237, 1976.

15. Vogler WR, Chan Y-K: Prolonging remission in myeloblastic leukaemia by tice-stain Bacillus Calmette-Guerin. Lancet 2: 128, 1974.
16. Ochoa JJ: Alkylating agents in clinical cancer chemotherapy. Ann NY Acad Sci 163:281, 1969.
17. Delmonte L, Jeskes TH: Folic acid antagonists in cancer chemotherapy. Pharm Res 14: 91, 1962.
18. Ellison RR, Burchenal JH: Therapy of acute leukemia in adults. J Chron Dis 6: 44, 1957.
19. Greenwald ES: Chemotherapy of Cancer. Medical Examination Publishing Co., New York, 1973, pp. 199–212.
20. Gec TS, Yu KP, Clarkson BD: Treatment of adult acute leukemia with Arabinosyl Cytosine and Thioguanine. Cancer 23: 1019, 1969.
21. Neuros N et al: The Vinco alkaloids. In Advances in Chemotherapy, vol. 5, Ed. A. Golden and F. Hawshing, Academic Press, New York, 1964, p. 133.
22. Djerassi I, and Jung SK: Methotrexate and citrovorum factor rescue in the management of (non-Hodgkin's lymphomas) childhood lymphosarcoma and reticulum cell sarcoma. Cancer 38: 1043–1051, 1976.
23. Johnan IS et al: The Vinco alkaloids. A new class of oncolytic agents. Cancer Res 23: 1390, 1963.
24. O'Bryan RM et al: Phase II evaluation of adriamycin in human neoplasia. Cancer 32: 1, 1973.
25. Barron M et al: Daunorubicin in the treatment of acute myelocytic leukemia. Lancet 1: 330, 1969.
26. Gilladoga AC, Manuel C, Tan CTC, Wollner N, Sternberg SS, Murphy ML: The cardiotoxicity of Adriamycin and Daunomycin in children. Cancer 37: 1070, 1976.
27. Rosen G, Suwansirikul S, Kwon C, Tan C, Wu SJ, Beattie EJ, Murphy ML: High dose Methotrexate with Citrovorum Factor Rescue and Adriamycin in childhood sarcoma. Cancer 33: 1151, 1974.
28. Durant JR, Lessner HE: Development of four drug BCNU combination chemotherapy regimens. Cancer 32: 277, 1973.
29. Schein P, Kahn R, Gorden P et al: Streptozotocin for malignant insulinomas and carcinoid tumor. Review of eight cases and review of the literature. Arch Intern Med 132: 555, 1973.
30. Luce JK et al: Clinical trials with the antitumor agent 5 (3,3,dimethyl-1-triazeno) imidazole-4-carboxamide (NSC 45388). Cancer Chemother Rep 54: 119, 1970.

# THE IMMUNOTHERAPY OF CANCER*

MICHAEL A. SILVERMAN, M.D.,
PETER W. A. MANSELL, M.D.

## THE THEORY OF IMMUNE SURVEILLANCE

A great deal of research is being done at present to determine the therapeutic usefulness of immunologic manipulations in the patient with cancer. The rationale for the use of immunotherapy in man is based on a number of *in vivo* and *in vitro* observations both in man and animals suggesting the importance of the immune system in host defense, not only against organisms, but also against malignancy. A major theory derived from these observations, although rather controversial, is that of immune surveillance, which was proposed by Thomas and Burnet (1).

This theory proposes that the host's immune system acts as a natural defense against cancer. There are three basic tenets to this theory:

1. Normal cells transform into malignant cells with the formation of antigens that are not present in normal cells.
2. These new antigens can be recognized as foreign by a competent host-immune system, thus inducing a specific immune response.
3. This immune response, elicited by the tumor antigens, can then cause destruction of the malignant cells.

A number of clinical observations seem to support the theory:

1. The highest incidence of cancer in man is seen in the very young and the very old (2,3). In the former case the immune system is not fully developed, and in the latter it is beginning to fail.

---

*Supported, in part, by *NIH-NCI* Grant No. CA14395-05

2. The incidence of malignancy is increased in patients with immunodeficiency disorders (4). Patients with Burton's type agammaglobulinemia, a disease characterized by defects in humoral immunity, show a 10,000-fold increase in leukemia compared to the normal population. Patients with ataxia telangiectasia and the Wiscott-Aldrich syndrome, diseases characterized by combined immune deficiencies, have an incidence of cancer 10,000 times that of the normal population, most commonly malignant lymphoma.

3. Following renal transplantation patients who are on various immunosuppressive regimes have a markedly higher incidence of neoplasia than normal (5). These include epithelial tumors of the skin, cervix, and lip, in addition to lymphomas, often of the CNS.

4. It is also known that cancer in man can occasionally undergoes spontaneous regression, suggesting that the host-immune system rejected the tumor (6,7). The malignancies most commonly reported to regress spontaneously are malignant melanoma, neuroblastoma, hypernephroma, and choriocarcinoma. Other malignancies described as undergoing spontaneous regression include testicular, ovarian, colon, breast, bone, soft tissue, and bladder tumors.

5. A frequent clinical observation is that of a very long latent period between the appearance and treatment of the primary tumor, and recurrence of the disease. This latent period can be as long as 20 years in some cases, and is most often seen in tumors of the breast and malignant melanoma. The presumed explanation for this is that the malignant cells have been latent in the body since the appearance of the primary but have been under the control of the immune system, and only when this control breaks down as the result of intercurrent illness or some other stress does the tumor recur.

6. It is frequently seen that the same type of tumor may pursue widely differing courses in different patients. For instance, one patient may have an extremely slowly growing tumor while another, with the same histological type of tumor, may have very rapidly progressing disease, reminiscent of fulminant infection in the preantibiotic era. One of the reasons for this could well

be differences in the ability of the host-immune defenses to deal with cancer.

7. Many investigators have reported on the finding of malignant cells in the peripheral blood; however, there is seldom a correspondingly high incidence of metastatic disease in those patients with circulating tumor cells (8). Although the occurrence of blood-borne metastases depends on a large number of factors, not all of which are immunological, there is mounting evidence that antibodies are capable of destroying circulating tumor cells, thus preventing their attachment to endothelium and their establishment as metastases.

Certain pathological observations also appear to support the concept of immune surveillance (9,10). Patients in whose tumors marked lymphocytic infiltration is seen have a more favorable prognosis than those whose tumors do not show lymphocytic infiltration. The malignancies that seem to show a more favorable prognosis when lymphocytic infiltration is seen histologically include carcinoma of the breast, stomach, colon, and cervix, and malignant melanoma, neuroblastoma, and choriocarcinoma. The same observation is also true for macrophage infiltration of tumors. Thus patients with well-marked macrophage infiltrates tend to have a better prognosis than if no macrophages are seen. In animal tumor systems it has been shown that the number of macrophages in a tumor is inversely proportional to the frequency of metastases; also, other parameters of immune responsiveness, such as antibody mediated immunity, seem to correlate with tumor macrophage content. Thus not only lymphocytes but also macrophages play a part in the host's immune response to tumor. There is, in fact, increasing evidence to suggest that the immune system is one of cooperation rather than compartmentalization—lymphocytes, macrophages and antibody working together, not separately—as had been thought formerly.

Studies in animal tumor models and in humans with malignancy also lend support to the theory of immune surveillance (11). Recently developed inbred strains of animals have enabled investigators to show rejection of transplanted chemically and virally induced tumors by the competent host immune system. In addition, studies in humans have provided evidence of cell-mediated immune mechanisms against autologous tumors as well as allogeneic, histologically similar, tumors. These antitumor responses have been demonstrated in all human tumors studied to date. An additional piece of experimental evidence in support of the importance of the host's immune system is the recently reported finding of blocking factors, which are discussed in detail below. Of great current interest is the finding of factors elaborated by the tumor itself, which appear to be able to combat the host's immune system, thus abrogating any antitumor effect the host might be able to mount.

The theory of immune surveillance, however, remains controversial and has been challenged by a number of authors (12). They point out that certain immunoincompetent animals, "nude" mice, fail to develop neoplasia despite treatment with oncogenic viruses or chemical carcinogens. However, nude mice are capable of producing antibodies that may be important, particularly in virally induced tumors. Other investigators have observed that the incidence of malignancy in sarcoidoses and leprosy (secondary immunodeficiency diseases) is not increased compared to the normal population. These investigators note that the malignancies most commonly seen in Wiscott-Aldrich syndrome (a primary immunodeficiency disease) and in renal transplant patients on immunosuppressive therapy are lymphomas and epithelial tumors, malignancies thought to be possibly associated with oncogenic viruses. These investigators feel that the occurrence of malignancy in these diseases may be related to impaired immunity to infectious agents, such as oncogenic viruses, rather than impaired immunity to neoplasia. This, however, does not seem to deny the importance of immune surveillance as a central mechanism since whether the immunity is against *de novo* cell-surface anitgens or cell-surface antigens induced by transforming viruses is a matter of little significance. Only time will tell if the concepts of immune surveillance will remain as the cornerstone of our present approach to cancer immunotherapy or whether alternative theories will radically change this approach.

## Nature of the Immune Response

At one time authorities held a simplistic concept of host immune defenses against tumor cells. Cell-mediated immunity (CMI) was thought to play the major role, with thymus-derived lymphocytes (T cells) killing the tumor cells directly by largely unknown mechanisms. On the other hand, humoral immunity, represented by antibody, was regarded as being of minor importance, and possibly antagonistic, acting as a factor capable of blocking lymphocyte response in solid tumors even though antibody was known to be cytotoxic in leukemia. Thus the immune system was compartmentalized CMI, by which was meant lymphocytes being "good," and antibody being "bad," in general. Recent studies have shown, not surprisingly, that the immune defense system is much more complex than was thought originally.

Apart from T cells many subpopulations of lymphocytes have been identified. Complicated interactions have now been demonstrated between T cells and thymus-independent lymphocytes (B cells), nonimmune lymphocytes, or null cells, have been identified and shown to be capable of killing cells in the presence of specific antibody (13-15). T-cell actions are now known to be influenced by T helper and suppressor cells whose independent and interdependent actions seem to be responsible for the "fine tuning" of the cellular immune system. Complex deficiencies in all, or any, of these sytems could explain the imbalances seen in patients with malignant disease.

Macrophages have long been neglected as important mediators of antitumor immunity (16,17). In terms of numbers, cell for cell, macrophages are much more powerful killers of malignant cells than are lymphocytes. Moreover, an activated macrophage is capable of differentiating nonspecifically between malignant and normal cells, killing the abnormal and leaving the normal intact. Macrophages can also kill malignant cells in the presence of cytophilic antibody and are important in the production of antibody itself by acting as a processing cell for antigen (18). Many of the immunologically active agents discussed in detail later, such as *Bacillus* Celmette Guerin (BCG) and *Corynebacterium parvum* exert their action primarily as a result of being macrophage activators.

Antibody, originally considered unfavorable in terms of the patient, is now known to play an important part in the defense of the host against blood-borne tumor cells (19). Without this circulating defense mechanism it is likely that tumor cells in the peripheral blood would find it much easier to survive and subsequently to become implanted on the endothelium and form metastases. As has been mentioned, antibody interacts with immune cells in a number of situations to produce cell killing (20). Interestingly, the humoral immune system also appears to have its own inbuilt regulation system, as does the cellular system. It has long been known that patients with chronic infectious diseases produce antiantibodies, that is, antibodies directed specifically against their own gammaglobulin; the same occurs in cancer. This appears to be the mechanism for unblocking the system by neutralizing excess amounts of antibody that may remove (or bind with) free antigen, forming immune complexes that block the action of immune cells. Thus it can be seen that what started out as a simple concept has now become a fascinating and complicated one, with many cellular and humoral factors interrelating and providing their own self-regulating systems. The proper study of this system now demands extremely sophisticated methodology, some of which is discussed later.

### Why Does the Immune Response Fail?

In the face of such a complex defense mechanism the enigma is why a tumor ever develops, or if once developed, why it continues to grow and kill the patient. In man little, if anything, is known about the causation of cancer, whereas in animals many agents, chemical, viral, and physical, are known causes (21). In animals the antigens found on the surface of the malignant cells are easily recognized by the host's immune defenses. In man, on the other hand, these neoantigens are weak as compared to those found in animals or to bacterial antigens. It is thought, therefore, that these relatively weak antigens are only capable of eliciting a weak response. Perhaps more important than the strength of the response is the fact that it may well take longer to arise than a response to a strong antigen. Therefore, while the response is building up to an effective level, the tumor may have the opportunity to grow to a size, which, although only a few cells in magnitude, the immune response is still unable to affect.

Once a tumor has grown beyond a critical size, whatever that may be, several factors may come into operation to protect it from the host's immune system (22-24). As a tumor grows, the center of the mass becomes relatively inaccessible, so far as outside influences are concerned, and although in large tumors the center may become hypoxic, or even necrotic, there will remain a zone of cells that are perfectly viable but to which host cells cannot penetrate. As a tumor grows it sheds into the surrounding environment and the circulation an increasingly large amount of antigen, either as a result of cell death from natural causes or following immunological or therapeutic attacks. This antigen load can act in one of two ways to protect the tumor, CMI can be abrogated by large amounts of circulating antigen, and antibody can be neutralized in the circulation, forming antigen–antibody complexes. It is well known that patients with cancer can develop immune-complex disease, or nephrotic syndrome. If kidney biopsies are done in these cases it is not unusual to find immune complexes composed of antigen–antibody or even antibody–antibody, in the case where anti–antibody is being produced. Apart from antigen, it is now thought that tumors are capable of secreting into the circulation factors that can block immune defenses, but the exact nature of these factors is not known. Quite apart from these effects of a growing tumor is the fact that all tumors do not consist of uniformly similar cells, but of mosaics of cells that are different not only morphologically but also in function, biologic potential, and biochemical and immunological characteristics. This being the case, the body is presented not with one antigen to mount an immune response against but a large number, thus diluting the response further. Furthermore, there is evidence that during the lifetime of a tumor the antigens may be modulated and that the antigenic pattern of a primary may not necessarily be the same as that of its metastasis. Hence the body's immune defenses are presented with an enormous task.

Added to all this is the existence of: (1) antiantibodies, which while largely regulatory in nature, may also block specific antibody in some circumstances and (2) blocking antibody, which by masking antigenic sites may diminish the effectiveness of CMI (25).

Although helper and suppressor T cells are generally considered to assist the action of T cells, there are also abnormal helper and suppressor cells, which may further diminish whatever effective immune response there is (26).

There is a still further mechanism that tends to abrogate the host's immune defense against tumors and the well-meaning efforts of the doctor. So far as is known all available methods of cancer therapy are more or less immunosuppressive. This is certainly true of radiotherapy, chemotherapy with cytotoxic drugs and steroids, and to a somewhat lesser extent, surgery (27). A great deal of work has been done on this aspect of cancer therapy, and the effects are well documented. They are dose-related and vary in intensity and length of duration, nevertheless, there is no doubt that the very act of trying to cure a tumor may significantly depress the individual's ability to defend himself against that tumor. However, though this may be true, it should not lead to therapeutic nihilism since, in spite of the side effects, well-managed treatment should be designed so that the benefit in terms of the reduction of tumor mass far outweighs any effect of immuno-suppression. An area of very great research interest is that concerned with ways to protect the individual from the deleterious effects of treatment while preserving the benefits. Also, it is to be hoped that as the various ways in which a tumor escapes immune attack are better understood, it will become possible to devise ways of overcoming them.

## THE EVALUATION OF IMMUNE FUNCTION IN THE TUMOR-BEARING HOST

One of the problems with immunotherapy, which has been practiced since the early years of the century, has always been that the scientific evaluation of cause and effect has been difficult. The result of this has been that, until very recently, most attempts at immunotherapy, while apparently producing some effect in some instances, have provided little more than anecdotal material because of the inability on the part of the investigators to assign the supposed effect to the immunotherapy given with any degree of certainty. The realization that monitoring methods were necessary and that in experimental animals the demonstration of immune reactions to tumors was relatively simple led to the development of a number of *in vivo* and *in vitro* assays.

The most common method for the measurement of *in vivo* immune competence in man is the cutaneous delayed hypersensitivity test (28). An intradermal injection of a very small amount of a standardized antigen is given to an individual, and the resulting flare and induration are measured at standard intervals, usually 24, 48, and 72 hours. The presence of a response indicates that the individual had encountered the antigen previously and is capable of mounting a hypersensitivity reaction to it. The response is cell-mediated in type and depends on the function of T cells and macrophages. Numerous antigens are available for use, but those most commonly used are *Candida,* Mumps, purified protein derivative (PPD), and Streptokinase–Streptodornase (SKSD, Varidase). One of the most common and probably most useful measurements of delayed hypersensitivity is the dinitrochlorobenzene (DNCB) reaction (29). In this test a minute amount of the substance is applied to the surface of the skin for sensitization, and the individual is challenged 14 days later with standard amounts of the reagent. A positive test indicates capability for sensitization to a new substance, namely, the hapten DNCB, which combines with skin protein, followed by a delayed reaction. There is some evidence to suggest that the ability to become sensitized to DNCB and mount a reaction to it correlates with a relatively good prognosis. As far as the other, so-called standard, antigens are concerned in cancer, the evidence is much less clear. If a patient is negative with respect to a whole battery of antigens, he may then be termed "anergic," and this state is often seen in the later stages of malignant disease of all types, particularly diseases of the reticuloendothelial system, such as Hodgkin's disease (30). However, it is usually possible to predict with reasonable accuracy those patients who will be anergic without doing the test. One thing is certain; there is no point at all in doing these, or any other tests of immune competence, only once. The only real usefulness of these tests is to watch changes when they are done sequentially throughout the course of the disease, and in this way some meaningful information may be gained. As a general rule, immune competence declines as the disease advances (31). However, there are many other factors that may impair immune competence, such as age, stress, malnutrition, and infection, as well as treatment with cytotoxic drugs, steroids, radiotherapy, anesthesia, and surgery, which may all operate in the patient with cancer. All such factors must be borne in mind when assessing immune function in cancer patients.

Early attempts to assess immune competence in a more specific way by skin-testing patients with preparations of their own or other histologically similar tumors have not been generally successful. Obviously, there is a great need for a specific measurement of immunity against the patient's tumor, but this is not yet available, although there have been a number of claims made for it. Various *in vitro* tests of nonspecific and specific immune competence in patients with cancer have also been developed (31). The simplest method is to perform an absolute lymphocyte count on the patient's peripheral blood (32). Studies in patients with malignant melanoma and Hodgkin's disease have suggested that low initial lymphocyte counts indicate a worse disease prognosis. Some groups feel that the determination of numbers of peripheral circulating T lymphocytes by E-rosette formation is an important assay of immune competence (33). A number of reports have indicated that low T cell counts correlate with a worse prognosis and a more advanced stage of disease. Decreased levels of T lymphocytes have been described in a wide range of cancers, in particular, squamous-cell cancer of the lung, esophagus, and head and neck. *In vitro* T cell activity can be assessed by a number of methods, including blastogenesis, migration inhibition (MI), mixed lymphocyte culture (MLC), and cytotoxicity assays (31). The blastogenesis assay is a convenient test of the nonspecific activation of lymphoid cells by the plant mitogens phytohemagglutinin (PHA) and concanavalin-A (ConA) or of the specific activation of lymphoid cells by tumor antigens (34). The tests quantitate DNA synthesis by lymphocytes ("responder cells") after cultivation in the presence of mitogens or antigens. Various authors have attempted to correlate the response to PHA with the stage and course of the disease, but the results have been disappointing. The direct migration inhibition assay and the mixed leukocyte culture assay have also been used to study T lymphocyte function in patients with cancer. Despite early reports suggesting that these assays correlate with the prognosis and clinical course of the patient with cancer, many investigators have found that the usefulness of these tests is limited in the case of the patient.

Assays of cytotoxicity attempt to measure the direct killing effect of peripheral blood lymphocytes on monolayers of tumor cells in tissue culture (36). For technical reasons it is seldom possible to test a patient's lymphocytes against his own tumor, since it is not possible to establish all tumors in tissue culture. However, it is usually possible to test against established cell lines of allogeneic tumor cells. The obvious disadvantage of this method is that it is not clear whether the characteristics of allogeneic cultured cells remain constant or whether they correspond with those of the particular patient's tumor. These tests assess cell killing in one of two ways, either visually by simply

counting the remaining target cells attached to the glass after incubation with the lymphocytes for a standard time, or by counting the
release of an isotope from the labeled target cells after incubation. A
number of isotopes are used, the most popular at present being chro-
mium $Cr^{51}$ (37). Unfortunately, the results of cytotoxicity assays are
variable, nonspecific reactions are known to take place, and cross
reactions are frequent. These cross reactions occur not only between
patient's lymphocytes and tumor cells of types other than the patients'
tumor, but between normal lymphocytes and tumor cells of various
types, thus making the test difficult to interpret and unreliable. Results
also vary from center to center, clouding the issue even further. The
colony inhibition assay, which is closely related to cytotoxicity assays,
is subject to similar criticism. Quantitative measurement of B cells is
possible by counting the fluorescing cells after labeling with a fluorescent anti-Ig that must be polyvalent (38). Some assessment of B cells
number and function can be obtained by incubating peripheral blood
lymphocytes with Pokeweed Mitogen (PWM) and counting DNA replication after labeling with tritiated thymidine, as with PHA and ConA.
However, PWM is not a specific B-cell mitogen, and the results are
not straightforward.

The measurement of monocyte/macrophage activity is more complex even than measuring lymphocyte function (39). There are methods
for evaluating phagocytosis, chemotaxis, and intracellular killing of
organisms, but none of these are particularly useful. Two methods that
may have some application in the future are the simple measurement
of peripheral blood monocytes, which can be done very accurately
using a fluorescent antimonocyte serum and passing the cells through
a machine that counts only those cells that shine in the dark. The other
method that has aroused some interest recently is an indirect one in
that it measures the amount of an opsonin which is present in the
blood. Without this, opsonin (RF) macrophages are not able to function effectively. The amount of RF is diminished in the blood of patients with malignant disease, and the amount of reduction appears to
relate to the tumor burden and thus to prognosis to some extent.

The measurement of the humoral response to tumor has now been
recognized as important. This is usually attempted by measuring circulating immunoglobulin levels but is quite useless except in such diseases as multiple myeloma, where huge increases of monoclonal gam-

maglobulins are seen. Another possible application of this method is in the measurement of an alpha-2-globulin, which some investigators have reported to be elevated in cancer, but the significance of this is not clear. No useful information is to be gained by the general measurement of gammaglobulin fractions, since the changes and amounts involved in the immune response to malignancy are altogether too subtle. More meaningful assays of antibody responses can be obtained by the use of specific fluorescent methods and by measuring complement-dependent antibody cytotoxicity in much the same way as lymphocyte cytotoxicity is measured. Neither of these two methods has gained general acceptance, although the former has provided very valuable information on the antigens present on the surface and in the interior of tumor cells. Other "humoral" factors that are sometimes measured include the various components of complement, acute-phase reactants, and so on, but their place in making up the picture is still under investigation.

The problem of measuring immune function in malignant disease is essentially that the available methods are unreliable, difficult to interpret, complex, and, therefore, not easily reproducible and extremely time-consuming. Until better methods are available it is probably true that this exercise should only be attempted by those well equipped to do it and that the interpretation should, at best, be guarded.

## FETAL ANTIGENS

Various antigens have been described in malignant disease that are similar to those found in normal fetal tissue (40). In normal adult tissue the antigens present on the cell surface differ from those found in fetal tissue of the same type. What is presumed to have happened, in the case of some malignant diseases, is that the adult antigens have reverted to the fetal type or that the fetal antigens have become derepressed as a result of the neoplastic process. There are two main examples of this phenomenon.

The so-called $\alpha$-fetoprotein in malignant hepatoma is an interesting substance as it represents a true tumor antigen, but as it only occurs in approximately 50% of hepatoma patients, its diagnostic usefulness is strictly limited. The other compound in this class is carcinoembryonic antigen (CEA), which is a fetal antigen described in carcinoma of the colon. This antigen has some application in the care of the cancer patient, since if it is measured sequentially the varying levels have some correlation with tumor load. Thus if a patient has a high level before operative removal of the tumor and this subsequently drops to normal, one can be reasonably sure that the operation removed all, or most, of the tumor. If the level remains low, this usually indicates that there is no recurrence, whereas if the level rises, there should be high clinical suspicion of a recurrence. Unfortunately, a high level does not necessarily mean that there is a recurrence, nor does a low level mean that there is no recurrence; hence, merely measuring the CEA does not absolve the physician from following the patient properly. High CEA levels can also be seen in other conditions such as cancer of the breast and lung and even in some normal conditions. It is probable that CEA represents a family of compounds rather than a single substance, and much work remains to elucidate its significance.

## IMPORTANT CONSIDERATIONS FOR SUCCESSFUL IMMUNOTHERAPY

Studies in animals with experimental tumors have shown that manipulation of the immune system can produce prolonged survival and even cure in some circumstances. These therapeutic results generally correspond with an increase in measurable immune reactions against the tumor. Following these experiences in animals similar techniques have been tried in man with varying degrees of success. Before considering these methods, however, it is necessary to mention some basic criteria for successful immunotherapy:

1. The tumor burden should be a low as possible (41). This is one of the basic criteria for any form of adjuvant therapy of cancer, whether immunotherapy or chemotherapy. It has repeatedly been shown in animals and man that while an individual with a great deal of tumor may be able to mount an antitumor immune response, that response is extremely unlikely to be effective in the presence of a large tumor load. For this reason it is worth considering bulk-reducing procedures such as surgery and chem-

otherapy before turning to immunotherapy, always bearing in mind that these other modalities may be immunosuppressive.

2. The patient should be immunocompetent (42). There is obviously no point in trying to use immunotherapy if the patient is incapable of mounting an immune response. On the other hand, it can be argued that the very reason for using immunotherapy is to restore immune responsiveness to an otherwise anergic host. Bearing these two apparently conflicting points in mind, a possible rationale exists for the use of two types of immunotherapy: (a) one that will restore immune competence—possibly transfer factor, immune RNA, thymosin, or other methods discussed later—and (b) a specific form of immunotherapy designed to direct the host's immunological attention to the specific tumor—for instance, the use of autologous or allogeneic cell vaccines.

3. There should generally be contact between the immunological agent and the tumor cells (43). In the case of BCG this is best seen when the agent is injected into the lesion, whereas in the case of a systemically administered agent it has to be possible for the effector cells of the host's immune system or the humoral factors to attack the malignant cells effectively.

4. The dose of immunotherapy must be carefully formulated. Too little will be ineffective but, more importantly, too much may not only be dangerous because of toxic reactions, but may even cause enhancement of tumor growth (44). Immunotherapeutic agents can be just as toxic to the patient as cytotoxic drugs if given unwisely. Severe side effects and death have been reported as a result of giving immunotherapy in the wrong doses to the wrong people. It goes without saying that immunotherapy should only be given under controlled circumstances where there are facilities for immune monitoring and the proper care of the patient. Immunotherapy is quite definitely not an "office procedure" for the general practitioner.

## METHODS OF IMMUNOTHERAPY

There are three methods of immunotherapy (45,46): (1) passive, (2) adoptive, and (3) active. Each method of immunotherapy can further be subdivided into specific and nonspecific. Passive immunotherapy is really only of historic interest (47). In the early 20th century, immunotherapy was practiced by means of transfusing serum into the patient from either an immunized animal or from a human being who appeared to be cured of cancer. Although there were some reports of success, this method is no longer practiced, and there seems no reason to revive it. There are still occasional reports of spontaneous remissions in leukemia patients after transfusion. Of peripheral interest, since it crosses the boundaries between passive immunotherapy and chemotherapy, are the attempts by some investigators to link chemotherapeutic drugs with specific antibody. The rationale is that the antibody will enable the drug to be directed to the malignant cell where it will be released in high concentration *in situ*. The drug most often used is chlorambucil. Apart from a few isolated reports, this technique has not been particularly successful.

Adoptive immunotherapy is the technique of transferring from one individual to another either immunologically active cells or substances so that the recipient adopts the immunological profile of the donor (48). There are basically four ways of doing this. The first was originally reported by Nadler and Moore and consists in the transfer of peripheral blood white cells from one individual to another (49). The donor can be either a normal person or one who has been cured of cancer, or the technique of cross-transplant cross-transfusion can be used. In this technique two patients with the same type of tumor are matched for blood-group compatibility, and tumor from one is removed and transplanted into the other, and vice versa. After 14 days, when the immune response should be maximal, each patient is bled of one unit of blood for 10 successive days. The blood is separated, the red cells are returned to the donor, and the white cells are transfused into the other patient. Thus white cells from patient A who had been immunized with tumor from patient B are returned to B. In theory, these white cells will then kill the tumor. Success has been reported in a few cases, particularly in patients with melanoma and sarcoma, but the method is not widely used. One of the drawbacks is the tediousness of the technique for both patient and physician. There have been a number of reports in which the donor of the sensitized cells has been animal rather than human, usually a pig; again, this method has not gained much popularity. Refinements of the general technique exist in which specific populations of cells are transfused, for instance, thoracic-duct lymphocytes, but more work needs to be done on this method. Adoptive transfer of immunity can also be achieved using three subcellular agents derived from immunologically competent cells. These agents are transfer factor, thymosin, and immune RNA.

Transfer factor is a low-molecular-weight (mol. wt. 10,000) extract of human peripheral lymphocytes, first isolated by Lawrence 20 years ago (50). This extract is capable of transferring specific, and probably nonspecific, cell-mediated immunities of the donor to the recipient. Transfer factor is DNase- and RNase-resistant and has been demonstrated to increase macrophage chemotaxis and enhance certain lymphocyte responses to plant mitogens. Traditionally, transfer factor has been used in patients with obvious and profound T-cell dysfunctions, including lepromatous leprosy, chronic mucocutaneous candidiasis, coccidiomycosis, and the Wiscott-Aldrich syndrome. The risks of transfer factor are unknown, but probably quite small. Transfer factor is nonimmunologic, and there are no reports of allergic reactions. There have been a few cases of an autoimmune hemolytic anemia, a lymphoproliferative syndrome, and even suppression of immune mechanisms in patients receiving transfer factor treatment, but these reports are at best anecdotal. Transfer factor is administered by intramuscular injection and may produce burning at the site of local injection. Initial studies with transfer factor in patients with solid tumors demonstrated that skin-test reactivity could be transferred from donor to recipient after the administration of transfer factor. These findings led to a number of investigations using transfer factor in the treatment of patients with various forms of cancer, which are, however, preliminary (51–53). It is suggested that transfer factor may be able to transfer specific immunity against osteogenic sarcoma from appropriate donors (e.g., household contacts and relatives) to patients with osteogenic sarcoma (54). Whether transfer factor will be of clinical benefit in this or any other type of malignant disease as adjuvant therapy is not yet known.

Thymosin is a soluble product of calf thymus (55). It is capable of restoring skin allograft rejection and has the ability to elicit graft versus host (GVH) disease in neonatally thymectomized mice. Thymosin also stimulates tissue growth and induces the appearance of T-cell markers in bone-marrow cells. It apparently has an effect on T-cell differentiation. Thymosin Fraction V isolated by Goldstein consists of 12 poly-peptides with molecular weights ranging from 12,000 to 14,000. Thymosin has been shown to reconstitute cell-mediated immunity in several patients with immunodeficiency disease. Thymosin is administered intramuscularly. There have been no reports of major toxicity associated with the administration of this substance. Preliminary trials of its use in malignant disease are under way, but no significant reports have yet appeared (56).

Immune RNA is a high-molecular-weight substance derived from lymph-node and splenic lymphocytes of specifically immunized animals, usually sheep (57). Immune RNA is capable of transferring both CMI and humoral immunity to the recipient, and there has been a great deal of excellent experimental work done on this subject, particularly by Pilch and his associates. Clinical trials of this substance are so far confined to its use in late stage renal adenocarcinoma, and some striking results have been reported. There is general agreement that this agent is of interest but that the clinical experience needs to be expanded (58).

Active immunotherapy is the area in which there is most interest at present. Active immunotherapy can either be specific or nonspecific (59-63). Specific active immunotherapy refers to the use of tumor cells or tumor-cell extracts. The tumor cells may be fresh autologous cells, cultured cells, or allogeneic cells, or homogenates of cells, or cell membrane fractions. Recently there has been renewed interest in the use of tumor antigens. When whole cells are used as the vaccine they are rendered incapable of further division while remaining viable, by being irradiated or in some instances by being treated with glutaraldehyde. In early experiments when this was not done some instances of autotransplantation with subsequent growth of the transplant were recorded, but this is obviously not a problem with subcellular vaccines. However, little success has been reported unless whole cells have been used. Because cell-surface antigens are generally regarded as being weak in human cancer, some attention has been paid to the possibility of enhancing their antigenicity. There have been attempts to do this by attaching to the cells strong antigens such as rabbit gammaglobulin in much the same way as one might try to break immunological tolerance, or by attaching to the cell antigenic viruses such as influenza virus. These experiments are interesting but have not been confirmed as effective. Another possible reason for the inefficiency of the anti-tumor response is that the antigen may be masked, for instance, by sialic acid residues on the cell membrane. To unmask antigens in this situation, cells have been treated with the enzyme neuraminidase, prepared from *Vibrio cholerae*. This is a successful technique in animals but has thus far not been very effective in man (64). Obviously, the use of pure tumor antigen would be the best way to immunize a patient specifically. Although a great deal of work has been done on the isolation of such antigens, no entirely satisfactory preparations have yet been produced. Specific active immunotherapy is theoretically an attractive method of immunotherapy, and there is no doubt that specific immune reactions have been recorded in patients after active immunization. The very nature of the method, however, somewhat restricts its use since fresh autologous cells are the best immunogen, in the absence of pure antigen. As has been discussed earlier, the use of cultures or allogeneic cells may not be ideal because of antigenic differences between these cells and the patient's own tumor. Cell homogenates and cell-membrane fractions have not proved effective. Since the supply of fresh cells is limited in any particular case, so is the number of times a patient can be immunized, even if the cells can be satisfactorily stored. Much work continues to be done in this field, and it is probable that the best application of immunotherapy will be a combination of specific active immunotherapy with immune restoration using either transfer factor, thymosin, or immune RNA.

Nonspecific active immunotherapy refers to the use of the immune adjuvants (65,66). There are numerous such agents, many of which are effective, but most have the disadvantage that they are toxic, which restricts their use. The general theory behind their use is that by generally stimulating the body's immune system, so also will the body's immune response to the tumor be increased *pari passu*. What appears to happen, in principle, is that the agents act as general activators of macrophages for the most part and also act on the various members of the T-cell system, thus generally alerting the immune defenses. It is of interest that there have been recent reports of cross reactivity between BCG antigens and melanoma antigens, in particular the cytoplasmic antigen, so that in this case nonspecific immunotherapy may be more specific than was originally thought.

The BCG vaccine is a live attenuated bacillus derived from bovine tubercle bacilli (67-71). The vaccine is not standardized, and much controvery exists as to whether the particular substrain or the method of preparation affects its antitumor activity. The vaccine contains large clumps of dead bacilli and subcellular debris, as well as viable myco-bacteria, which usually make up less than 5%. A number of substrains of BCG have been used such as Pasteur, Tice, and Glaxo. It is ad-ministered in a number of ways, either in direct contact by injection into tumor nodules or instillation into the pleural cavity, or system-atically by intradermal injections using a Heaf gun or Tine plate or by scarification (72). BCG is also given orally and is effective when given this way; indeed, this is the method used by its originators to protect children against tuberculosis. Two mechanisms for the antitumor ac-tivity of BCG have been suggested. Early studies indicate that contact between activated macrophages and tumor cells may account for much of the nonspecific antitumor activity of BCG. *Bacillus* Calmette Guerin may also stimulate systemic tumor-specific immunity by concentrating thymus-dependent lymphocytes within the tumor site and mediating the activity of macrophages that process tumor antigens. A number of complications have been described after therapy with BCG (73). These include local abscess formation, a flu-like syndrome, nausea, malaise, granulomatous hepatitis, disseminated BCGosis, and anaphylactic re-actions, with even a few reports of death. The theoretical possibility of tumor enhancement after BCG treatment exists and has been sug-gested in a few studies in which patients with melanoma treated with BCG have had a decreased disease-free interval compared to concom-itant controls. A nonviable extract of the attenuated BCG organisms left after extraction of phenol-killed bacteria with methyl alcohol, is MER (methanol extraction residue) (74). MER has been shown to have the ability to increase the antitumor activity in mice prophylactically. Methanol extraction residue is currently being evaluated in a number of human tumor systems, as are other BCG related preparations in which BCG cell walls are attached to oil droplets—the so-called Ribi vaccine. Preparations from other strains or mycobacteria are also un-der investigation.

Various strains of Corynebacterium have also been shown to act as reticuloendothelial stimulants (75-77). The formaldehyde-killed vac-cines in particular of *C. parvum* and *C. granulosum* have the ability to increase antitumor activity in a number of animal tumor models.

*Corynebacterium parvum* can increase the production of IgM and IgG antibody to various antigens and apparently can activate both the classical and alternate pathways of complement. *Corynebacterium parvum* has been shown to activate the reticuloendothelial system. In animal tumor systems, intravenous or intraperitoneal *C. parvum* given before implantation of tumors can inhibit tumor growth. Based on these animal studies, *C. parvum* has been administered to humans by both intravenous and subcutaneous routes. The most common complications include shaking chills and fever after intravenous administration and local tenderness and swelling after subcutaneous injection. *Corynebacterium parvum* is currently being evaluated in a large number of human tumors, it is generally considered to be of very little use unless given intravenously. Other biological agents used as immunotherapy include Coley's toxin, pertussis, and vaccinia. Many successes were reported for Coley's toxin in the early years of the century, and it is still under investigation in some centers.

Levamisole is the levorotatory form of tetramisole, a synthetic antihelminthic (78,79) Levamisole does not stimulate immunologic responses to excessive levels, nor does it have an effect on the responses of immunologically intact individuals. It is primarily active in the immunorestoration of deficient host mechanisms, hence it is not an immunostimulator in conventional terms, but an immunomodulator (80). The exact mechanism of the action of levamisole on the immune response is unknown, but accumulating data suggest an influence on T lymphocytes and T–B lymphocyte interaction. Evidence also points to an effect of levamisole on the macrophage–monocyte, which in turn regulates lymphocyte activity. Levamisole apparently restores depressed cell-mediated immunity without significantly affecting humoral mechanisms and increases the cyclic GMP level while decreasing the cAMP level of T-lymphocytes. Levamisole can be adminstered orally or parenterally, but is only used in the oral form in man (81). It is absorbed rapidly from the alimentary tract and peak plasma levels are seen 2–4 hours after administration, with a plasma half-life of 4 hours. The primary site of levamisole metabolism is the liver. Within 3 days approximately 70% of levamisole is excreted in the urine unchanged or as metabolites. The side effects of levamisole include anorexia, irritability, nervousness, nausea, fatigue, skin rashes, and reversible agranulocytosis. Levamisole has been shown to have antitumor activity in animal models. Preliminary trials in man have shown some activity in lung cancer; one of the interesting points to emerge from this particular study was that levamisole is only effective when given in the proper dose, 2.5 mg $\cdot$ kg$^{-1}$ of body weight. This is usually given on 2 consecutive days per week. A recent report has also indicated some effect in breast cancer, but this is unconfirmed. There is great interest in this substance because of its ease of administration, chemical nature, and relative lack of side effects. Levamisole should not be given to patients with autoimmune diseases such as rheumatoid arthritis because of the increased incidence of agranulocytosis.

Other agents such as tilorone, pyran copolymer, and the polysaccharide glucan are under investigation as immune adjuvants. The first two are very toxic, while the third has the advantage of being nontoxic (82,83). It is too early to comment on their effectiveness. Another method of immunotherapy, though not generally recognized as such, is the use of topical agents in the treatment of skin malignancies. The most commonly used of these is 5-FU cream, which is used in the treatment of superficial basal and basosquamous-cell carcinomata, actinic keratoses, and lentigo maligna. In these cases 5-FU does not act primarily as a cytotoxic agent, but as a hapten and elicits a delayed hypersensitivity reaction, in much the same way as DNCB.

One of the major roles of nonspecific active immunotherapy is to boost and maintain the specific response seen after immunization of the patient with autologous irradiated cells, allogeneic cells, or antigen. Ordinarily the specific response will decline after about 21 days so that the patient has to be reimmunized to maintain the response. This may not always be possible, because of lack of cells for instance. If nonspecific immune adjuvants such as BCG or levamisole are given simultaneously, this decline in immune response can often be postponed or prevented altogether.

## THE ADMINISTRATION OF IMMUNOTHERAPY

Immunotherapy can be given in one of a number of different ways (84–86):

1. LOCAL INJECTION OF TUMORS. Lesions of malignant melanoma and breast cancer have been shown to regress in a high number

of cases after local injections of BCG and other agents. In some cases noninjected lesions also regress.

2. PROPHYLACTIC IMMUNOTHERAPY. It has been reported that prophylactic vaccination with BCG of a population of children against tuberculosis reduced the incidence of acute lymphatic leukemia, but these studies have not been confirmed by other investigators. Our knowledge of immune manipulation must be greatly increased before considering any prophylactic immunotherapy of a normal patient population in the hope of decreasing the subsequent incidence of cancer.

3. SYSTEMIC ADMINISTRATION OF IMMUNOTHERAPY AS ADJUVANT THERAPY. Adjuvant therapy is defined as that therapy given after all clinically detectable disease has been removed. A number of encouraging but unconfirmed investigations have suggested that this may be the most important area of immunotherapy in man. Adjuvant studies are now in progress in colon, breast, and lung cancer and in leukemia, malignant melanomas, and sarcomas. The results of these are eagerly awaited.

4. SYSTEMIC IMMUNOTHERAPY FOR ADVANCED CANCER. The studies applying immunotherapeutic modalities in patients with widespread cancer have as a rule yielded dismal results when given in combination with other modalities of therapy or alone. These results are predictable based on animal data. The outcomes of these and other studies were reported at a conference in late 1976. With the exception of a handful of reports, all the studies were negative.

## CONCLUSIONS

Since the end of the 19th century the science of immunology has made extraordinary advances, bringing in its wake the newer subspecialty of tumor immunology. Although immunotherapy experiments in human cancer began at about the turn of the century, there was a long hiatus in the 1930s and 1940s, after the first flush of enthusiasm had died down. In a classical review Woglom wrote in 1929 that "nothing is to be hoped for in the treatment of cancer from immunotherapy." We have come a long way since then, but many of the old questions still remain.

There have been numerous clinical trials on leukemia (ALL, AML), malignant melanoma, sarcomas, and carcinomas. Isolated success has been reported, and this has stimulated a great renewal of interest. The area of most promise appears to be the use of immunotherapy as an adjuvant and, although there is no general agreement as to which is the best method, many trials are now in progress. It seems likely that no one method of immunotherapy will emerge as the best and that combination treatment, as in chemotherapy, will be the answer. Thus a patient may first have to have his immune responsiveness restored nonspecifically with an agent such as transfer factor, thymosin, or immune RNA. Next he will have to be specifically immunized against his tumor and later have his immunity boosted and maintained by the use of a nonspecific agent such as BCG, *C. parvum,* or one of the others in this group. It may well be that immunotherapy programs will have to be as painstakingly individualized as most other forms of therapy. It is certain that great attention will have to be paid in planning to concomitant chemotherapy, radiotherapy, and surgery. The immunotherapist is now part of the multidisciplinary oncology team, and it is likely that this exciting field of research and development will play an increasingly important role in cancer therapy in the future.

## REFERENCES

1. Burnet FM: The concept of immunological surveillance, Prog Exper Tumor Res 13: 1, 1970.
2. Peto R, Ive FS, Lee PN et al: Cancer and aging in mice and men. Brit J Cancer 32: 411, 1975.
3. Stutman O: Cell mediated immunity and aging. Fed Proc 33: 2028, 1975.
4. Kersey JH, Spector BD, Good R: Primary Immunodeficiency Disease and Cancer. The Immunodeficiency—Cancer Registry, Int J Cancer 12: 333, 1973.
5. Penn I: The incidence of malignancies in transplant recipients. Transplant Proc 7: 323, 1975.
6. Everson TC, Cole WH: Spontaneous regression of cancer, Preliminary report Ann Surg 144: 366, 1956.
7. Cole WH: Spontaneous regression of cancer: The metabolic triumph of the host? Ann NY Acad Sci 230: 111, 1974.
8. Salisbury AJ: The significance of the circulating cancer cell. Cancer Treat Rev 2: 55, 1975.

9. Black MM, Opler SR, Speer FD: Survival in breast cancer cases in relation to the structure of the primary tumor and regional lymph nodes. Surg Gyn & Obstet 100: 543, 1955.

10. Martin RF, Beckwith JB: Lymphoid infiltrations in neuroblastoma. Their occurrence and prognostic significance. J Pediat Surg 3: 161, 1968.

11. Schwartz RS: Another look at immunologic surveillance. New Eng J Med 293: 181, 1975.

12. Prehn RT: Immunostimulation of the lymphodependent phase of neoplastic growth, J Natl Cancer Inst 59: 1043, 1977.

13. Perlmann P, O'Toole C, Unsgaard B: Cell-mediated immune mechanisms of tumor cell destruction. Fed Proc 32: 153, 1973.

14. Cerottini J, Brunner KT: Cell medicated cytotoxicity, allograft rejection. Advan Immunol Tumor Immunity 18: 67, 1974.

15. MacDonald HR, Bonnad GD: A comparison of the effector cells, involved in cell mediated lympholysis and antibody dependent cell-mediated cytotoxicity, Scad J Immunol 4: 129, 1975.

16. Lohmann W, Mathes ML: Induction of macrophage mediated cytotoxicity. In Immunobiology of the Macrophage. Ed. D. S. Nelson. Academic Press, New York, 1976, p. 464.

17. Mansell PW, DiLuzio NR, McNamee R, Rowden G, Proctor JW: Recognition factors and nonspecific macrophage activation in the treatment of neoplastic disease. Ann NY Acad Sci 277: 20, 1976.

18. Basten A, Mitchell J: Role of macrophage in T cell-B cell collaboration in antibody production. In Immunobiology of the Macrophage. Ed. D. S. Nelson. Academic Press, New York, 1976, p. 45.

19. Lewis MG: Circulating humoral antibodies in cancer. Med Clin N Amer 56: 481, 1972.

20. Saal JG, Rieker EP, Hadan M, Riethmuller G: Lymphocytes with T cell markers cooperate with IgG antibodies in the lysis of human tumor cells. Nature 265: 158, 1977.

21. Melief CJM, Schwartz RS: Immunocompetence and Malignancy. In Cancer: A Comprehensive Treatise on Etiology, Chemical and Physical Carcinogenesis. Ed. F. F. Becker, Plenum Press, New York 1975, p. 121.

22. Wind APP, Nairn, RC, Rollad JM et al: Lymphocyte anergy in patients with carcinoma. Brit J Cancer 28: 108, 1973.

23. Occhino JC, Glascow AH, Cooperband SR et al: Isolation of an immunosuppressive peptide fraction for human plasma. J Immunol 110: 685, 1973.

24. Alexander P: Escape from immune destruction by the host through shedding of surface antigens: Is this a characteristic shared by malignant and embryonic cells? Cancer Res 34: 2077, 1974.

25. Hellstrom I, Hellstrom KE, Sjogren HO et al: Serum factor in tumor free patients cancelling the blocking of cell-mediated tumor immunity. Int J Cancer 8: 185, 1971.

26. Gershon RK, Mokyr MB, Mitchell MJ: Activation of suppressor T cells by tumor cells and specific antibody. Nature 250: 594, 1974.

27. Hersh EM, Freirich EJ: Host defense mechanism and their modification by cancer chemotherapy. *In* Methods of Cancer Research IV. Academic Press, New York, 1968, p. 355.

28. Eilber FR: Sequential evaluation of general immune competence in cancer patients: Correlation with clinical course. Cancer 35: 660, 1975.

29. Catalona WJ: Quantitative dinitrochlorobenzene contact sensitization in a normal population. Clin Exp Immunol 12: 325, 1972.

30. Young RC, Gorder MP, Haynes HA, Levita VT: Delayed hypersensitivity in Hodgkin's Disease: Study of 103 untreated patients. Am J Med 52: 63, 1972.

31. Hersh EM, Mavligit GM, Gutterman JU: Immunodeficiency in cancer and the importance of immune evaluation of the cancer patient. Med Clin N Amer 60: 623, 1976.

32. Lee YT et al: Delayed cutaneous hypersensitivity and peripheral lymphocyte counts in patients with advanced cancer. Cancer 35: 748, 1975.

33. Potvin C et al: Thymus derived lymphocytes in patients with solid malignancies. Clin Immunol Immunopath 3: 476, 1975.

34. Golub SH: Host immune response to human tumor antigens. *In* Cancer. A Comprehensive Treatise. Ed. F. F. Becker. Plenum Press, New York, 1975, p. 259.

35. Mavligit GM, Hersh EM, McBride CG: Lymphocyte blastogenesis induced by autochthonous human solid tumor cells: Relationship to stage of disease and serum factors. Cancer 34: 1712, 1974.

36. Hellstron KE, Hellstrom I: Lymphocyte-mediated cytotoxicity and serum activity to tumor antigens. Adv Immunol 18: 209, 1974.

37. Puche JG, Canevari S, Fossati G, Porta GD, Vezzoni P: Complement—dependent serum cytotoxicity of cancer patient studied by $^{51}$Cr release assay on human cancer lines. Tumori 63: 97, 1977.

38. Rabellino E, Colon S, Grey HM, Unanue ER: Immunoglobulin on the surface of lymphocytes I. Distribution and quantitation J Exp Med 133: 156, 1971.

39. Snyderman R, Mergenhagen SE: Chemotaxis of Macrophages: *In* Immunobiology of the macrophage. Ed. D. S. Nelson, Academic Press, New York, 1976, p. 323.

40. Alexander P: Foetal "antigens" in cancer. Nature (Lond.) 235: 137, 1972.

41. Mathe G., Pouillant P, Lapeyraque F: Active immunotherapy of L1210 leukemia applied after the graft of tumor cells. Brit J Cancer 23: 814, 1968.

42. Hersh EM, Gutterman JU, Mavligit GM, McCredie KB, Bargen MA, Matthews A, Freireich EJ: Serial studies of immunocompetence of patients undergoing chemotherapy for acute leukemia. J Clin Invest 54: 101, 1974.

43. Hanna MG, Jr, Snodgrass MJ, Zbar B, Rapp HJ: Histopathology of tumor regression after intralesional injection and mycobacterium bovis IV: De-

velopment of immunity to tumor cells and BCG. J Nat Cancer Inst 51: 1897, 1973.

44. Hellstrom KE, Hellstrom I: Immunologic Enhancement of Tumor Growth. *In* Mechanisms of Tumor Immunity. Wiley, New York, 1977.

45. Bluming AZ: Current status of clinical immunotherapy. Cancer Chemotherapy Reps 59: 901, 1975.

46. Proctor JW, Lewis MG, Mansell PW: Immunotherapy of cancer: An overview. Can J Surg 19: 12, 1976.

47. Wright PW, Hellstrom KE, Hellstrom IE, Berstein, ID: Sero-therapy of malignant disease. Med Clin N Amer 60: 607, 1976.

48. Fefer A, Einstein AB, Jr, Chever MA: Adoptive chemoimmunotherapy of cancer in animals. Ann NY Acad Sci 277: 492, 1976.

49. Nadler SA, Moore GE: Clinical immunologic study of malignant disease: Response to tumor transplant and transfer of leucocytes. Ann Surg 164: 482, 1966.

50. Lawrence HS: Transfer Factor: Advan Immunol 11: 195, 1969.

51. Silverman MA, Meltz MA, Sorokin C, Glade PR: Effects of transfer factor in Waldenstrom's macroglobulinemia and multiple myeloma. *In* Transfer Factor: Basic Properties and Clinical Applications. Ed. M. S. Ascher, A. A. Gottlieb, C. H. Kirkpatrick. Academic Press, New York, 1976, p. 633.

52. Lo Buglio AL, Neidhart JA: A review of transfer factor immunotherapy in cancer. 34: 1563, 1974.

53. Krementz ET, Mansell PW, Hornung MO et al: Immunotherapy of malignant disease: The use of viable sensitized lymphocytes or transfer factor prepared from sensitized lymphocytes. Cancer 33: 394, 1974.

54. Levin AS, Byers VS, Fudenberg HH et al: Osteogenic Sarcoma: Immunologic parameters before and during immunotherapy with tumor specific transfer factor. J Clin Invest 55: 487, 1975.

55. Goldstein AL, Guha A, Zatz MM, Hardy MA, White A: Purification and biological activity of thymosin, a hormone of the thymus gland. Proc Nat Acad Sci 69: 1800, 1972.

56. Shafer LA, Goldstein AL, Gutterman JU, Hersh EM: In vitro and in vivo studies with thymosin in cancer patients. Ann NY Acad Sci 277: 609, 1976.

57. Deckers PJ, Pilch YH: RNA mediated transfer of tumor immunity: A new mode for the immunotherapy of cancer. Cancer 28: 1219, 1971.

58. Pilch YH, Fritze D, De Kernion JB, Ramming KP, Kern DH: Immunotherapy of cancer with immune RNA in animals and cancer patients. Ann NY Acad Sci 277: 592, 1976.

59. Mathe G, Amiel JL, Schwarzenberg L, Schneider M, Cattan A, Schlumberger JR, Hayat M, De Vassal F: Active immunotherapy for acute lymphoblastic leukemia. Lancet i: 697, 1969.

60. Powles RL: Immunotherapy for acute myelogenous leukemia using irradiated and unirradiated leukemia cells. Cancer 34: 1558, 1974.

61. Rosato FE, Miller E, Rosato E, Broun A, Marc K, Wallack K, Johnson

J, Moskowitz A: Active specific immunotherapy of human solid tumors. Ann NY Acad Sci 277: 332, 1976.

62. Stewart THM, Hollingshead AC, Harris JE et al: Immunochemotherapy of Lung Cancer. Ann NY Acad Sci 277: 436, 1976.

63. Wallack MK, Steplewski Z, Koprowski H, Prato E, George J, Hulihan B, Johnson J: A new approach in specific active immunotherapy cancer 39: 560, 1977.

64. Bekesi JG, St. Arneault G, Holland JF: Increase of leukemia L1210 immunogenicity by vibrio cholerae neuraminidase treatment. Cancer Res 31: 2130, 1971.

65. Mastrangelo MJ, Berd D, Bellet RE: Critical review of previously reported clinical trials of cancer immunotherapy with nonspecific immunostimulants. Ann NY Acad Sci 277: 94, 1976.

66. Milas L, Withers R: Nonspecific immunotherapy of malignant tumors. Radiology 118: 211, 1976.

67. Bast RC, Jr, Zbar B, Borsos T, Rapp HJ: BCG and cancer. N Eng J Med 290: 1413, 1974.

68. Morton DL, Eilber FR, Holmes EC, Hunt JS, Ketcham AS, Silverstein MS, Sparks FC: BCG immunotherapy of malignant melanoma: Summary of a seven year experience. Ann Surg 180: 635, 1974.

69. Nathanson L: Use of BCG in the treatment of human neoplasm: A review. Sem Oncol 1: 337, 1974.

70. Zbar B, Rapp HJ: Immunotherapy of guinea pig cancer with BCG. Cancer Res 34: 1532, 1974.

71. Gutterman JU, Mavligit G, Reed R: Immunology and immunotherapy of human malignant melanoma: Historical review and perspective for the future. Sem Oncol 2: 155, 1975.

72. Bornstein RS, Mastrangelo MJ, Sulit H: Immunotherapy of melanoma with intralesional BCG. Nat Cancer Inst Monogr 39: 213, 1973.

73. Aungst CW, Sokal JE, Jager BU: Complications of BCG vaccination in neoplastic disease. Ann Int Med 82: 666, 1975.

74. Robinson E, Bortal A, Cohen Y, Haas R: Preliminary report on the effect of methanol extraction residue of BCG (MER) on cancer patients. Brit J Cancer 32: 1, 1975.

75. Woodruff MF, Boak JL: Inhibitory effect of injection of corynebacterium parvum on the growth of tumor transplants in isogeneic hosts. Brit J Cancer 20: 345, 1966.

76. Israel L, Edelstein R: Nonspecific immunostimulation with c. parvum in human cancer. Paper presented at the Symposium of Immunological Aspects of Neoplasia. M. D. Anderson Hospital and Tumor Institute, Houston, Texas, 1974.

77. Israel L: Clinical results with corynebacterium parvum. *In* Investigations and Stimulation of Immunity in Cancer Patients. Ed. G. Mathe. Springer, New York, 1974, Vol. 1, p. 486.

78. Symoens J, Rosenthal M: Levamisole in the modulation of the immune response: The current experimental and clinical state. J Reticuloendothelial Soc, 21: 175, 1977.
79. Verhaegen H, De Cree JJ, De Cock W, Vergruggen F: Levamisole and the immune response. New Eng J Med 289: 1148, 1973.
80. Chirigos MS, Pearson JW, Pryor J: Augmentation of chemotherapeutically induced remission of a murine leukeumia by a chemical immunoadjuvant. Cancer Res 33: 2615, 1973.
81. Oettgen HF, Pinsky CM, Delmonte L: Treatment of cancer with immunomodulators. Corynebacterium parvum, levamisole. Med Clin N Amer 60: 511, 1976.
82. Munson AE, Munson JA, Regelson W, Wample GL: Effect of tilerone hydrochloride and congeners on reticuloendothelial system tumors and the immune response. Cancer Res 32: 1397, 1972.
83. Mansell PW, Rowden G, Hammer CM: Clinical experiences with glucan: In Progress in Cancer Research and Therapy. Ed. M. Chirigos. Raven Press, New York, 1978, Vol. 7.
84. Immunotherapy of cancer: Present status of trials in man. Progress in Cancer Research and Therapy. Ed. W. D. Terry, D. Windhorst. Raven Press, New York, 1978, Vol. 6.
85. Morton DL: Cancer immunotherapy: An overview. In Advances in Cancer Surgery. Ed. J. S. Najarian, J. P. Delaney. Grune and Stratton, New York, 1975 & 1976, p. 89.
86. Oettgen JR: Immunotherapy of cancer. New Eng J Med 297: 484, 1977.

# BREAST CANCER: A BRIEF REVIEW OF CURRENT CLINICAL CONCEPTS

CHARLES L. VOGEL, M.D., FRANCISCO TEJADA, M.D.

## THE MAGNITUDE OF THE BREAST-CANCER PROBLEM

One out of every 13–14 women born in the United States will experience cancer of the breast during her average lifetime of 72 years (1). It is estimated that in 1977 approximately 90,000 new cases were diagnosed and that 34,000 women died of the disease (1). Breast cancer is the leading cause of cancer-related death among women and is the commonest overall cause of death among women aged 40–44 (2). Although there has been a slight decline in mortality from breast cancer over the past two decades, this decline has been modest (from 25.9 per 100,000 in 1939–41 to 24.7 per 100,000 in 1964–66) (3).

## EPIDEMIOLOGY AND ETIOLOGY

Hormonal, environmental, and genetic differences among populations result in marked variations in risks for the development of breast cancer. Nulliparous women, those whose first pregnancy occurred later in life, those who did not breast feed, or those who have not undergone a surgical menopause prior to age 35 are at greater risk for the development of breast cancer (2).

White women are more commonly affected than blacks and other racial groups (4,5), and the disease is far more common among North American and Northern European women than in women from Latin America, Africa, and Japan (2).

There is a significantly increased risk of breast-cancer development among blood relatives of breast-cancer patients, and when it develops among daughters of probands it occurs at a mean age of 10 years younger than that at which their mothers were diagnosed (2). Women whose mother developed bilateral breast cancer premenopausally are at a ninefold greater risk of breast cancer than the general population (5).

Preexisting fibrocystic disease is still another risk factor, and patients who have already had cancer of one breast have a 10-15% probability of developing a second primary neoplasm in the opposite breast.

The role of estrogen, prolactin, and other hormones in the biology of human breast cancer has not been elucidated, but the topic has been recently reviewed and is the subject of intensive investigation (6).

It has been demonstrated that certain information in the RNA of human breast cancer is homologous to that of an RNA virus-induced mouse mammary tumor, thereby suggesting some viral role in the pathogenesis of human breast cancer (7).

## PATHOLOGY (2,8)

Twenty-two percent of all breast lesions turn out to be malignant neoplasms; 50% are diagnosed as fibrocystic disease, and the remaining 28% represent benign lesions, such as fibroadenomas, papillomas, lipomas, or traumatic disease of the breast.

The most common type of breast cancer, infiltrating ductal carcinoma, accounts for 74% of malignant neoplasms of the breast. Paget's disease and comedo, medullary, papillary, and lobular carcinomas together account for about 20% of malignant neoplasms. The remaining 6% include rare tumors such as fibrosarcomas and lymphosarcomas.

Infiltrating ductal carcinoma usually is accompanied by some degree of desmoplastic reaction (fibrosis), inducing contractures along the fascial planes of the breast, which often results in fixation of the neoplasm to the skin and chest wall with retraction of the nipple.

Breast cancer in males (9) includes any one of the histological types mentioned above and accounts for only 1% of all cancers in men. It appears at any age above 20 years, and the guidelines for therapy follow those for breast cancer in women.

## CLINICAL ASPECTS

### History (2)

Over 90% of women with breast cancer request medical attention after they notice a lump in their breast. Therefore, it is important to teach women self-examination of the breast, to be done at least once every month after the menses.

Other less common complaints include nipple or skin changes and axillary masses. Pain is not typically associated with a cancerous breast lump, but with benign fibrocystic disease or inflammatory breast masses. Nipple discharge, bleeding, and weight loss are not frequent complaints in breast cancer.

### Physical Examination (2)

Careful examination of the breasts with the patient in the sitting and supine positions should be carried out in all four quadrants of the breast, including the axillary extension. A careful search for nodes should be conducted in the inferior, lateral, and medial areas of the pectoralis minor and in the axillary and the supraclavicular areas.

*Diagnosis* Biopsy and histological examination is the only certain way to diagnose breast cancer, but it is important to exercise careful clinical judgment to avoid unnecessary biopsy of false lumps or masses. However, *it is mandatory to biopsy all new, discrete, three-dimensional breast masses.*

Of the various nonsurgical diagnostic techniques, mammography has proven most useful, and data from large screening programs (e.g., the Health Insurance Plan of New York) show that combined physical examination and mammography detected twice as many breast cancers compared to a nonscreened population (10).

More importantly in this study, a statistically significant advantage for "screened" as opposed to "unscreened" patients was found both in the percentage of cancer patients presenting with histologically negative lymph nodes at the time of surgery and also in patient survival (10).

In August 1976 the National Cancer Institute and the American Cancer Society published new "interim guidelines" for the use of mammographic screening based on the knowledge that there is at least a theoretical risk of cancer induction by routine mammography or xeromammography (11). A summary of the guidelines follows:

1. As with any x-ray examination, radiation dosage must be kept to the lowest dose consistent with good image quality. Newer low-dose techniques involve a dose of 1 rad or less.
2. For women of any age in which there is a suspected breast neoplasm, mammography is an accepted part of the complete diagnostic workup.
3. For asymptomatic women over 50 years of age, definite benefit from mammography in addition to physical examination has been demonstrated. Mammography is indicated as part of a regular screening program.
4. The sophisticated types of mammography currently available have not been in common use long enough to demonstrate definite benefit in reducing mortality for asymptomatic women aged 30–50 years. In younger women with evidence of being at special risk of breast cancer because of family history, reproductive history, prior breast cancer or other tumor, the benefits as well as the possible risks of x-ray mammography should be fully explained to the patient and the final decision made between her and the physician.
5. For women with a history of cancer in one breast, mammography of the contralateral breast should be done routinely.

In most large screening surveys, thermography has added little to the diagnostic accuracy of physical examination and mammography. Early detection by ultrasound and nipple-secretion cytology is still investigational.

Marker substances currently under investigation (e.g., CEA, urinary polyamines, HCG, casein, ferritin) thus far lack proof of clinical usefulness in detecting preclinical disease (12). The CEA procedure does appear to have some value in helping to monitor treatment in patients with metastatic breast cancer (13). Further research is needed in this area since current "early diagnosis" methodology can still only detect tumors containing at least $10^9$ tumor cells, and true "early diagnosis" must aim at detecting subclinical disease.

### Staging

Staging and its prognostic implications are of paramount importance in deciding on the appropriate therapy for each patient with breast cancer. Staging should be done before therapy is considered, and every effort should be made to investigate spread to regional lymph nodes and distant sites.

Over the years many staging systems have been advanced, and older literature citing survival statistics according to stage must take into account variations in these systems. Following is a brief synopsis of the newest staging system of the American Joint Committee (14):

*Stage 1.*   A freely movable primary tumor of less than 2 cm ($T_{1a}$) with histologically negative axillary lymph nodes ($N_0$) and no distant metastases ($M_0$).

*Stage 2.*   A freely movable primary tumor of greater than 2 cm ($T_2$) or a smaller tumor with histologic involvement of axillary lymph nodes ($N_1$) but with no distant metastases ($M_0$).

*Stage 3.*   A tumor greater than 5 cm ($T_3$) regardless of nodal or distant metastases is considered Stage 3. Less advanced primary tumors that are associated with histologically involved axillary lymph nodes that are fixed to each other ($N_2$) are also considered as Stage 3. For any of the above-listed tumor (T) or nodal (N) characteristics, there can be no distant metastases ($M_0$).

*Stage 4.*   Local tumors fixed to the chest wall or having associated satellite nodules ($T_4$), ulceration or skin edema (peau d'orange) or cases of inflammatory carcinoma ($T_5$) are considered as Stage 4 regardless of the status of regional lymph nodes or distant metastases. Homolateral supraclavicular nodes ($N_3$) or arm edema are likewise considered as Stage 4 regardless of T or M status. Any tumor with distant metastases ($M_1$) is also considered as Stage 4.

**Prognosis**

Untreated breast cancer has an overall survival rate from time of diagnosis to death of 20% at 5 years and less than 10% at 10 years (15). The use of radical mastectomy at Johns Hopkins Hospital before 1950 gave a 5-year survival rate of 47% and a 10-year survival rate of 30% (2). More recent studies show that those elements included in disease staging are important prognostic variables. Staging features such as tumor size, fixation to skin, pectoralis muscles, or chest wall, and the degree of axillary lymph-node involvement facilitate the differentiation between "good-" and "poor"-risk patients. Thus, while at least 65% of patients in Stage 1 can expect to be free of the disease after 10 years, only 40% of Stage 2 and 15% of patients who have more than four histopathologically involved lymph nodes are free of the disease (16).

Several other variables have been described as possible prognostic determinants, including histologic type, blood-vessel invasion, sinus histiocytosis, degree of tumor differentiation, and patient age or menopausal status. More recently, the presence of estrogen-receptor proteins in tumor tissue has been described as still another variable, independent of other known prognostic indicators (17).

Estrogen-receptor determinations were initially described as predictive tests for hormonal responsiveness in patients with breast cancer. Thus, of patients with metastatic breast cancer whose tumors contain cytoplasmic estrogen-receptor proteins, 60% might be expected to respond to some form of additive or ablative hormonal manipulation, while less than 10% of patients with negative estrogen receptor assays have hormonally dependent tumors (18).

Even when the disease becomes widely metastatic, certain factors can influence prognosis. Thus, if the dominant site of metastases is soft tissue rather than visceral, the likelihood of response to both hormones and chemotherapy is increased. It has been stated that responsiveness of bone disease to therapy is the worst, but this may only be a reflection of difficulties inherent in evaluation of response in predominant osseous disease. Indeed, many investigators feel that responsiveness of bone lesions falls between that of soft tissue and that of visceral lesions.

### Treatment

Only general guidelines for treatment at the time of initial diagnosis and clinical staging are mentioned here since the overall treatment plan for a patient with breast cancer should be decided in consultation with medical, surgical, and radiotherapeutic oncologists at the time that pathological staging is available.

## TREATMENT FOR OPERABLE STAGE 1, 2, AND 3 BREAST CANCER

After diagnostic biopsy has been carried out and the diagnosis of breast cancer has been established, radical mastectomy is still the most commonly employed, primary surgical treatment, with 88% 5-year survival for Stage 1 and 62% 5-year survival for Stage 2. With this type of surgery, at least 65–85% (1,16) of patients without neoplastic involvement of axillary lymph nodes will still be free of the disease at 10 years, but only 15–40% of those with involved nodes will remain free of the disease (16). More extensive surgical procedures such as the extended radical mastectomy have not improved cure rates (19).

Less radical surgical procedures are under investigation and, at the present time, modified radical mastectomy has replaced radical mastectomy as the preferred operation at our institution. One interesting study being done by the National Surgical Adjuvant Breast Program (NSABP) has not yet shown significant differences in distant relapse rates at 5 years between clinical Stage 1 patients treated with radical mastectomy, simple mastectomy plus postoperative radiation therapy, and simple mastectomy plus radiation therapy at the time of locoregional recurrence (20). The most recent NSABP study randomizes clinical Stage 1 patients to simple mastectomy or segmental mastectomy (lumpectomy) with or without radiation therapy. These important studies will take several more years to complete follow-up, and as controversy will continue until then, radical or modified radical mastectomy should still be considered the surgical treatment of choice.

Postoperative radiotherapy has been shown by the NSABP to decrease the number of local and regional recurrences in patients receiving a radical mastectomy for operable breast cancer but with no improvement in cure rates (21). Hence, there is no clearly demonstrated survival advantage to the use of postoperative irradiation as an adjuvant to surgery in the routine treatment of operable breast cancer.

Surgical adjuvant chemotherapy should be considered for patients with Stage 2 and 3 disease because of promising early results of controlled clinical trials (22,23) using either L-Phenylalanine mustard (L-PAM; Alkeran) or a combination of Cytoxan, Methotrexate, and 5-FU (CMF). In these studies, patients with involved axillary lymph nodes were randomized after radical or modified radical mastectomy to receive either chemotherapy or no chemotherapy, and in neither study was postoperative radiation therapy used.

Recent (1977) updates of the L-PAM and CMF studies continue to show significantly lower relapse rates among premenopausal patients receiving chemotherapy as compared with those not receiving chemotherapy (24,25). Among postmenopausal patients, however, no such differences are apparent 3 years postoperatively. At present there are many new controlled trials of various combinations of adjuvant chemo-, immuno-, radiation, and hormonal therapies under study, but results are not yet available. Until the results of these trials are completed, therapeutic decisions should be made after: (1) review of available preliminary results of possible benefits, (2) analysis of the potential risks and hazards of adjuvant therapies, and (3) discussion of both potential benefits and potential risks with the individual patient.

There are no data from large-scale, controlled clinical trials available on the use of adjuvant chemotherapy in patients with Stage 1 disease. Since there is an approximate 65–85% cure rate obtainable by standard surgical techniques and a potential risk of carcinogenicity from chemotherapeutic agents, the use of adjuvant chemotherapy in patients with Stage 1 disease should be approached with considerable caution and fully informed patient consent. The use of chemotherapy in such patients is not common practice at our institution.

## TREATMENT FOR INOPERABLE STAGE 3
## AND STAGE 4 DISEASE

The clinical management of these patients calls for the expertise of a coordinated oncologic team to individualize the treatment of the patient since surgery, radiotherapy, and hormonal and chemotherapy in some form of combined modality approach is usually the best initial treatment for the patient.

In general, radiotherapy is the mainstay of therapy for locoregional disease covering the area of the primary lesion and the axillary, supraclavicular, and internal mammary nodes. Sometimes a simple mastectomy is indicated after radiotherapy to remove large, bulky or ulcerated tumors, but its use should be individualized. Studies are being conducted to determine the best combination of treatment modalities for "inoperable" Stage 3 disease.

When breast cancer is metastatic to distant sites, systemic therapy is indicated. Classically, the first hormonal manipulation used would be oophorectomy for premenopausal patients and exogenous estrogen administration for postmenopausal patients. Both of these maneuvers could be expected to produce clinical improvement in 25–40% of patients so treated. Discussions of the role of other hormonal therapies such as adrenalectomy, hypophysectomy, androgens, progestational agents, Aminoglutethimide, and the new antiestrogens such as Tamoxifen, goes beyond the role of this brief overview (26–28). Today the predictive value of estrogen receptor assays has made the oncologist's choice of systemic therapies less empirical. Patients with estrogen-receptor positive tumors are likely (60%) to respond to hormonal manipulation; however, if a patient is found to have a tumor that does not contain estrogen receptors, it would be logical to bypass hormonal manipulation and proceed directly with cytotoxic chemotherapy (18), since the expected rate of response to hormonal manipulation would be less than 10%.

Chemotherapy for metastatic disease results in objective tumor shrinkage of 50% or better in over 50% of the patients. Responses last for an average of 8–10 months. Combination chemotherapy is clearly superior to single-agent therapy (29), and the most effective combinations usually include Cytoxan and 5-FU with either Methotrexate (the CMF regimen) or Adriamycin (CAF) (30). The use of such combinations in an adjuvant situation for locoregional disease is being prospectively studied, and preliminary results are encouraging, as previously noted.

# REFERENCES

1. American Cancer Society: Cancer facts and figures. American Cancer Society Publication, 1977.
2. Brennan MJ: Breast cancer. In Cancer Medicine, Holland JF and Frei E, III (eds.). Lea and Febiger, Philadelphia, 1973, pp. 769–1788.
3. Cutler SJ: Increasing incidence and decreasing mortality rates for breast cancer. Cancer 28: 1376, 1971.
4. Seidman H: Cancer statistics, 1976: A comparison of white and black populations. Ca—A Cancer Journal for Physicians 26: 2, 1976.
5. Petrakis NL: Genetic factors in the etiology of breast cancer. Cancer 39: 2709, 1977.
6. Kirschner MA: The role of hormones in the etiology of human breast cancer. Cancer 39: 2716, 1977.
7. Schlom J: Differences in mouse mammary tumor viruses. Cancer 39: 2727, 1977.
8. Fisher E: The pathology of invasive breast cancer. Cancer 36: 1, 1975.
9. Donegan WL: Carcinoma of the male breast. Arch Surg 106: 273, 1973.
10. Shapiro S: Evidence on screening for breast cancer from a randomized trial. Cancer 39: 2772, 1977.
11. Bailar JC, III: Mammography: A contrary view. Ann Int Med 84: 77, 1976.
12. Franchimont P: Simultaneous assays of cancer associated antigens in benign and malignant breast diseases. Cancer 39: 2806, 1977.
13. Steward AM: Carcinoembryonic antigen in breast cancer—Serum levels and disease progress. Cancer 33: 1246, 1974.
14. Robbins GF: Classification of breast carcinoma: Changing concepts. Int J Radiation Oncology, Biol Phys 2:1191–1200, 1977.
15. Bloom HJG: Natural history of untreated breast cancer. Brit Med J 2: 213, 1962.
16. Fisher B: Biological and clinical considerations regarding the use of surgery and chemotherapy in the treatment of primary breast cancer. Cancer 40: 574, 1977.
17. Knight WA, III: Estrogen receptor as an independent prognostic factor for early recurrence in breast cancer. Cancer Res 37: 4669, 1977.
18. McGuire WL, Ed.: Estrogen Receptors in Human Breast Cancer. Raven Press; New York, 1975.

19. Fisher B: The surgical dilemma in the primary therapy of invasive breast cancer: A critical appraisal. In Current Problems in Surgery. Year Book Medical Publishers, Chicago, Ill, 1970.
20. Fisher B: Comparison of radical mastectomy with alternative treatments in primary breast cancer. Cancer 39: 2327, 1977.
21. Fisher B: Post operative radiotherapy in the treatment of breast cancer. Ann Surg 172: 711, 1970.
22. Fisher B: L-Phenylalanine mustard (L-PAM) in the management of primary breast cancer. NEJM 292: 117, 1975.
23. Bonadonna G: Combination chemotherapy as adjuvant treatment in operable breast cancer. NEJM 294: 405, 1976.
24. Fisher B: L-Phenylalanine mustard (L-PAM) in the management of primary breast cancer. Cancer 39: 2883, 1977.
25. Bonadonna G: The CMF program for operable breast cancer with positive axillary nodes. Cancer 39: 2904, 1977.
26. Kennedy BJ: Principles of endocrine therapy. In Cancer Medicine. Ed. J. F. Holland and E. Frei, III. Lea and Febiger, Philadelphia, 1973, pp. 889–950.
27. Santen RJ: Kinetic, hormonal and clinical studies with aminoglutethimide in breast cancer. Cancer 39: 2948, 1977.
28. Kiang DT: Tamoxifen (antiestrogen) therapy in advanced breast cancer. Ann Int Med 87: 687, 1977.
29. Broder LE: Combination chemotherapy of carcinoma of the breast. Cancer Treat Rev 1: 183, 1974.
30. Smalley RV: A comparison of Cyclophosphamide, Adriamycin, 5-Fluorouracil (CAF) and Cyclophosphamide, Methotrexate, 5-Fluorouracil, Vincristine, Prednisone (CMFVP) in patients with metastatic breast cancer. Cancer 40: 625, 1977.

# MAJOR GASTROINTESTINAL MALIGNANCIES

RICHARD MANN-KAPLAN, M.D.

## COLORECTAL CARCINOMAS

Cancer of the colon and rectum strikes more Americans than any other cancer except skin cancer and takes the lives of more than any but lung cancer. This year 101,000 cases are expected in the United States, and half of these patients will die of the disease. The sexes are equally affected so that, though its incidence is lower than that of lung cancer in men and breast cancer in women, its overall incidence is higher than either. Two-thirds of patients are over the age of 50, but the cancer can be seen in patients in the second, third, and fourth decades of life.

The U.S. incidence rate has been little changed in the past several years after having risen rapidly through the 1940s. The incidence is similarly high in Great Britain and several other industrialized northern European nations but is considerably lower in southern Europe, Asia, and Latin America. There is a striking rough *inverse* correlation with gastric carcinoma.

### Etiology

A few high-risk groups can be identified, though these account for only a small fraction of overall incidence.

*Familial Polyposis* This is an hereditary, Mendelian dominant, syndrome. It is thus seen in many members of an affected family, and its identification in a new patient demands a workup of the entire family. Innumerable adenomatous polyps carpet the entire large bowel, developing after birth and usually manifesting in childhood or adolescence as bleeding or diarrhea. These small polyps individually seem to have no greater chance of malignancy than sporadic polyps of comparable size, but a 1% or so chance, multiplied by hundreds of polyps, yields a 100% certainty of malignancy, usually in the third or fourth decade of life.

Prophylactic proctocolectomy with ileostomy by age 20 is indicated. Some surgeons compromise by leaving the rectum intact and following the patient with very frequent proctoscopy with fulgeration of all polyps. In one series, polyps in the remaining rectum were frequently seen to regress following subtotal colectomy. However, leaving the rectum in place is inherently risky since as many as 59% may eventually develop invasive carcinoma.

*Gardner's syndrome* is a similar entity, also Mendelian dominant, in which colonic polyps are associated with benign mesothelial tumors such as osteomas of skull and jaw, lipomas, fibromas, desmoid tumors, and sebaceous cysts. *Turcot's syndrome* is the association of glioma or medulloblastoma with multiple polyposis. The therapy is the same.

However, *juvenile polyposis* is an unrelated entity and is not premalignant. Here the polyps are "inflammatory" with columnar epithelium, prominent mucus cysts, and an inflammatory infiltrate. The small bowel may be involved as well as the colon, and colectomy is not indicated.

Similarly, *Peutz-Jeghers syndrome* is not truly premalignant. The polyps are hamartomas of the small bowel, important because they may bleed, and rarely degenerate into malignancy. The syndrome is usually recognized by pigmented lesions on the lips, buccal mucosa, and digits. However, 5% of females with this disease may develop ovarian tumors.

**Individual Polyps**    The chance of malignancy depends on the type and size of the polyp. The previous figures for frequency of malignancy have had to be revised downward as smaller polyps are being identified and removed via the fiberoptic colonoscope. In any case, for the common *adenomatous polyps*, if the polyp is less than 1 cm in diameter, the chance of malignancy is <1%; if 1–2 cm, about 1.5%; 2–3 cm, at least 10%; and those >3.5 cm have a 30–50% chance. If there is a long stalk or pedicle, the chance of finding cancer is reduced.

The less common *villous adenomas* have a higher malignancy rate, 40% or more overall, with less relation to size, but they tend to be larger anyway. These lesions are usually recognizable by their soft, frond-like surface, friability, and tendency to bleed. They not infrequently cause a mucous rectal discharge and occasionally cause a severe watery diarrhea with resultant profound hypokalemia and dehydration. With some tendency to recur, even when benign, and their high malignant potential, surgical resection is the treatment of choice, rather than simple endoscopic polypectomy.

There is an expanding body of experience suggesting that endoscopic removal of adenomatous polyps found to harbor malignancy, but not invading through the muscularis (i.e., Dukes A), may be considered adequate treatment. If, however, the tumor invades the muscularis, surgical bowel resection must be carried out.

*Ulcerative Colitis* Classic ulcerative colitis carries an enormous risk of ultimate development of large-bowel cancer when the disease involves the entire colon diffusely (not when limited to the rectum or rectosigmoid) and when the disease is continuously active for 10 years or more (mean = 16 years). Under these circumstances the proportion of patients who eventually develop cancer may be as high as 45–57%. The tumors that develop are more frequently right-sided or in the transverse colon and generally carry a very poor chance for survival, in part because of differences identifiable pathologically (frequent multicentricity, greater invasiveness, and higher degree of anaplasia), and probably in part because of the difficulty in diagnosing this complication by symptoms or x-rays in the chronic ulcerative colitis patient.

Total proctocolectomy is the procedure of choice when cancer develops (because 52% are multicentric) and in addition must strongly be recommended for prophylaxis in the patient with pancolitis of more than 10 years of activity.

The degree of corresponding risk for the *Crohn's disease* patient is not as clear, but these patients seem to have a somewhat increased incidence of adenocarcinoma, less so than in ulcerative colitis.

*Ureterocolonic Anastomoses* Ureterocolonic anastomoses are also recognized to predispose to the development of carcinoma distal to the anastomosis.

This leaves the etiology of the disease in the majority of patients unaccounted for. A wealth of epidemiologic data, retrospective studies, and experimental animal work now point to the role of the Western diet and/or life-style in the endemic pattern of colon cancer in the U.S.

The following relationships seem to hold and, at the present time, primacy cannot be claimed for any single one:

1. The risk of colon cancer increases when a low-risk group (e.g., the Japanese) moves to a high-risk area (e.g., the U.S.).
2. Higher-risk populations tend to have diets lower in residue and fiber (leading to longer transit times) and higher in animal fat and protein and refined carbohydrates.
3. Low-risk groups tend to defecate several times a day, while the Western life-style tends to discourage this. With a slow transit time, carcinogens may be kept in contact with bowel mucosa longer, or less obvious elements of causation could be at work.
4. High-risk populations have higher proportions of anaerobic bacteria in their bowel flora and tend to have higher concentrations of secondary bile salts. Both tend to potentiate experimental chemical carcinogenesis in animals.
5. Numerous substances in our environment have served as experimental carcinogens or cocarcinogens for colon tumors in animals.
6. For some reason, the worldwide incidences of gastric cancer and colon cancer seem to be inversely related.

A synthesis of the above evidence does suggest dietary factors in the development of large-bowel cancer. Whether a change in the dietary habits of an individual could be expected to affect his risk is, however, controversial.


**Diagnosis**


*Screening* Routine annual proctoscopic examination of asymptomatic individuals, though vocally advocated for some time, is probably defunct as a public-health measure. The yield of invasive cancer not palpable by digital examination is about 0.1%. To identify one *potentially* curable tumor costs in the range of $70,000–100,000. In addition, personnel are not available to apply this technique on a population-wide basis.

However, *the Greegor test* utilizing Hemoccult® slides, 2 daily × 3 days on a high-residue, no-meat diet seems to accomplish the same purpose. That is, it seems to detect about the same number of asymptomatic patients with a colorectal cancer. The overall cost is only a fraction as great because the test does not require professional personnel. Hopefully, a major campaign for its use will be mounted.

If one of the six samples in the Greegor test is positive for blood, a full gastrointestinal workup is warranted because some source of blood loss (although sometimes only hemorrhoids) is found in 99%. That is, there is only a 1% false-positive rate. When compared to screening by other techniques, the false-negative rate appears very low also.

The *carcinoembryonic antigen* (CEA) is not useful as a screening test because its level is usually proportional to the stage of the tumor, with most clearly abnormal valves reflecting large lesions or the presence of metastases. Thus CEA is relatively poor at detecting the curable lesions. Its greatest value lies in its use as a tumor "marker" (see below).

*Signs and Symptoms*   The consistency of stool as it traverses the large bowel, the caliber of the bowel at the site of origin, and the growth pattern of the tumor together predict the presentation. In the cecum and ascending colon the caliber is large, the feces are liquid, and tumors tend to grow in a polypoid or fungating pattern; thus obstruction is rare. These tumors tend to be friable and bleed, but this bleeding is usually slow and prolonged, or the blood has time to darken prior to reaching the rectum so that the patient frequently fails to recognize it. Therefore, right-sided lesions present with anemia or with only vague, dull, poorly localized pain. Since the tumor may grow quite large prior to causing alarming symptoms, an abdominal mass may be present on examination.

On the other hand, in the left colon stool is more solid, the luminal caliber is smaller, tumors tend to grow more circumferentially, and it is a shorter distance to the rectum, so that left-sided lesions present with change in bowel habits, change in stool caliber, cramps, obstruction, or bright red bleeding which hasn't yet produced much anemia. When the tumor arises in the rectum itself, obstruction is not as frequent since tenesmus is such a prominent earlier symptom.

Finally, a proportion of patients present either with constitutional symptoms of a malignancy (anorexia, weight loss, malaise, poor activity tolerance, etc.), remote effects of cancer, or symptoms of distant metastases.

*Workup*   Although there has been a trend toward more proximal large-bowel cancer recently, still about 60% of adenocarcinomas arise in the rectosigmoid. Therefore, rectal examination and proctoscopy are, if anything, more important than *barium enema*. The barium enema is in fact unreliable for evaluation of lesions within the pelvis. In addition, the barium enema as routinely done may miss small lesions or *any* lesion in the redundant areas of the bowel (e.g., in the sigmoid and near the flexures). An *air-contrast barium enema* detects 40% more polyps and 20% more carcinomas and should be done whenever cancer is suspected, unless the routine barium enema is diagnostic. Care should also be taken to visualize the entire bowel including the cecum before pathology is ruled out.

*Fibreoptic colonoscopy* has been an important advance in the handling of polyps (which can now be excised and examined instead of just followed) and the diagnosis of smaller carcinomas. This technique too has blind spots (just past each angulation) but is complementary to air-contrast barium enema. Colonic lavage for exfoliative cytology via fiberscope has been investigated in some centers, particularly for high-risk patients.

In addition to the "routine" blood tests and chest x-ray, both IVP (to assist the surgeon in anticipating retroperitoneal spread) and liver scan are recommended preoperatively. A positive liver scan or chest x-ray for metastatic disease or a positive biopsy of a suspicious node could, of course, change the surgical approach.

**Carcinoembryonic Antigen**   Carcinoembryonic antigen levels will be elevated (>2.5 mg/n liter) in 19–40% of patients with tumor localized in the bowel and in 96% of patients having distant metastases. A large number of common conditions also elevate CEA: COPD, or just cigarette smoking without much COPD, cirrhosis, ulcerative colitis, Crohn's disease, uremia, or chronic renal disease, peptic ulcer disease, pancreatitis, and cancers of the pancreas, stomach, lung, breast, ovary, bladder and other organs. Therefore, CEA is only an effective screening test for *advanced* cancer. However, it does have usefulness pre- and postoperatively and in long-term follow-up.

An elevated CEA that falls to normal postoperatively implies a complete resection and therefore a better prognosis. It may take CEA 1–2 months to reach its lowest level following successful surgery. A CEA that does not fall to normal, or falls but then rises again, implies a recurrence at a local or distant site that will manifest itself clinically usually 3–6 months later.

Some surgeons thus recommend a "second look" laparotomy for a rising CEA without demonstrated recurrence on clinical and radiologic studies. My own feeling is that it is only a rare patient whose recurrent cancer will prove resectable at such a "second look" and that the procedure should be reserved for the younger patients and most aggressive cancer surgeons.

## Pathology and Staging

The vast majority of colorectal carcinomas are, of course, adenocarcinoma of various degrees of differentiation, often staining positively for mucin. There has been a trend toward more proximal sites of origin in the U.S. for the past couple of decades, but it still remains true that the majority are digitally palpable or visible by proctosigmoidoscopy. Approximate distribution is:

16% Cecum, ascending colon, and hepatic flexure
11% Transverse colon and splenic flexure
11% Descending colon
21% Sigmoid colon
41% Rectum

Several variations of the Dukes classification have been used. One useful one (modified from Astler and Coller) is as follows:

| | | APPROXIMATE 5 YEAR SURVIVAL |
|---|---|---|
| A | Limited to mucosa and submucosa | 75–80% |
| B1 | Through muscularis, but not as far as serosa | 50–60% |
| B2 | To, or through, serosa with negative nodes | 25–30% |
| C | Positive nodes | 20% |
| D | Distant metastases | 5% |

In general, tumors of the rectum of a given stage have a slightly worse prognosis than equivalent lesions of the colon. This may be because the surgical margin of resection around them is necessarily smaller. In any case, careful second-look laparotomy studies have shown that tumors of the rectum usually recur first locally—either alone or together with liver metastases.

In recent years, animal model tumors and careful analysis of human solid tumors have advanced the concept of "micrometastases"—tiny invisible distant metastases that are already present at the time of apparently curative resection of the primary tumor and that account for the later appearance of metastatic disease. In animals, these micrometastases can be eradicated by chemotherapy at the time of primary tumor removal, and this has been the rationale behind use of chemotherapy, for example, after mastectomy. Such *"adjuvant chemotherapy"* has not been definitively tested in colorectal cancer yet, but the high rate of *local* relapse in rectal tumors may have to be taken into account in planning such studies.

### Therapy

*Polyps* See discussion under "Etiology" for an approach to handling adenomatous polyps without invasive malignancy. An adenomatous polyp with a short stalk or with an invasive cancer, despite apparently complete removal endoscopically, should be treated as the usual adenocarcinoma, that is, with a bowel resection taking adequate margins of normal bowel. The same is true of all villous adenomas. The main controversy concerns the necessity of surgery for a malignant adenomatous polyp with a long stalk and no invasion of the submucosa.

*Surgery* This is probably advisable even when metastatic disease is present except in the very poor operative risk, since expected survival is usually at least a year or two and surgery may be expected to reduce or prevent serious problems with bleeding and/or obstruction.

*Radiation* It is not generally appreciated that radiotherapy has a rather good record of *palliation* of symptoms of tenesmus, pain, and bleeding in rectal carcinoma (although the *cure rate* after radiation therapy is only 5–10%). This has led to studies of the role of preoperative radiation in this disease. These have demonstrated that the Dukes stages of treated patients are lower (better) than expected in untreated patients. Whether this means that treated patients with, say, Dukes B lesions will survive as long as patients with "natural" Dukes B lesions remains to be seen. The only category of patients where a survival advantage has shown up so far is in the patient where the tumor is so low in the rectum that A-P resection must be done. This is the group in which, as pointed out in the "Pathology" section, it is most difficult to achieve adequate surgical margins and in which local recurrence is very frequent, so that preoperative radiation may well be aiding control.

*Chemotherapy* For 20 years, 5-FU has been the only single agent to yield as many as 20% objective responses (>50% shrinkage of measurable tumor for longer than a month) of recurrent or metastatic colorectal cancer. Recent studies have compared the various dosage schedules and shown that a ''loading'' type course is more effective than weekly injections and that oral 5-FU responses are less frequent and of shorter duration. Many chemotherapists now feel that a regimen of 12–15 mg/kg/day for 5 days in a row, once a month is the best standard regimen. The toxicity is usually quite mild leukopenia, gastrointestinal upset, or stomatitis. Most patients tolerate this schedule very well.

Other active agents for palliation include Mitomycin-C, BCNU, CCNU, Methyl-CCNU (the latter is experimental), and Methotrexate.

Until recently, no combination proved superior to 5-FU alone. However, there is now ample evidence that Methyl-CCNU + 5-FU + Vincristine is superior in that it induces 30–40% objective responses (7). Unfortunately, the median duration of such responses is only about 5 months (as with 5-FU alone). Therefore, the impact on survival of the whole treated group (responders and nonresponders) is minimal.

In addition, the combination of Methyl-CCNU + 5-FU + Vincristine is much more toxic and difficult to handle than 5-FU alone and should only be used by experienced chemotherapists. The ultimate role for this combination, if any, may be as a surgical adjuvant treatment regimen (see below).

Metastases limited to the liver may also be treated by several other techniques. Since the blood supply of malignant liver tumors is derived largely from the hepatic artery while the arterial supply to the normal liver is primarily from the portal vein, ligation of the former may induce necrosis of hepatic malignancies. Unfortunately, this is usually very transitory and incomplete. Infusion of chemotherapy directly into the hepatic artery is advocated in some centers, but its real value is unknown since it is such a cumbersome procedure that all the published series are selected and no controlled trial has been done.

Other techniques under investigation include liver irradiation and 5-day constant IV infusions of high doses of 5-FU.

*Surgical Adjuvant Therapy* Because the prognosis for Dukes B2 and higher lesions is far from acceptable, and because of the patterns of failure outlined in the "Pathology" and "Staging" sections, colorectal cancer is one of the solid tumors where the combination of several modalities of therapy might be hoped to improve the cure rate.

Simple chemotherapy with 5-FU, FUdR, or ThioTEPA has been studied extensively. Although one "historically controlled" study (Li and Ross) claimed positive results, several well-controlled large-scale trials have failed to show a survival advantage to 5-FU used as a single agent (5,6). This evidence is so strong that it is not justified to use 5-FU for this purpose.

However, now that the three-drug combination of 5-FU + Methyl-CCNU + Vincristine has been shown to be more active, conceivably it will prove to be active enough to be useful as a surgical adjuvant. Several immunotherapeutic agents (BCG and MER–BCG) are being tested in the same way, but none of the controlled studies are far enough along to have yielded any conclusions.

Finally, as pointed out above, radiation may yet prove a valuable surgical adjuvant for rectal primaries, either pre- or postoperatively.


## ADENOCARCINOMA OF EXOCRINE PANCREAS


### General Considerations

Pancreatic carcinoma is now the fourth leading cause of cancer death in the U.S., with 20,300 new cases per year, virtually all of whom will die of the disease. Those aged 50–70 years are most frequently affected, and this malignancy is 2–3 times as common in males and appears to be increasing in black males.

The median survival after diagnosis is only 4–6 months, and many series report 90% of patients dead in 12 months. Slightly better results are being reported recently (see "Therapy" section).

Seventy percent of the cases involve the head, 20% the body, and 10% the tail. A surrounding area of pancreatitis is usual. Tumors arising in the body and tail have slightly shorter survivals and tend to metastasize earlier, presumably since they do not give rise to jaundice while still small.

Local extension of the tumor is the rule and, unfortunately, only a rare patient is a candidate for a "curative" resection. Invasion of the duodenum, common bile duct, superior mesenteric or splenic vessels, portal vein, regional lymph nodes, and regional nerves are all common. Distant metastases are to liver, peritoneum, lungs and pleurae, adrenals, bones, and spleen.

There is some evidence to link chemical exposure to pancreatic cancer and there is, in addition, a correlation with high-cholesterol diets and cigarette smoking.

It should be noted that *cystadenocarcinoma* is a rare pancreatic malignancy quite frequently cured by surgery and not to be confused with the more common malignancy discussed here.

**Symptoms and Signs**

Pain is often the presenting symptom and becomes a serious problem in 70–80% of patients. It is often ill-described at first and may have been present for several months or longer, but it eventually tends to evolve into an epigastric or hypochondriac dull, boring pain with or without back radiation, classically partially relieved by flexing the spine or bending over. Presumably for this reason it is often worst at night. Aspirin seems to have a disproportionate effectiveness compared to narcotics. In addition to "pancreatic pain," nonspecific bowel complaints are common.

Anorexia and weight loss (the latter is possibly also related to malabsorption) are nearly always present and usually marked.

Jaundice occurs in nearly all of the 75% of patients with lesions in the head of the gland but is usually not really "painless." True painless jaundice suggests more strongly carcinoma of the bile ducts or ampulla of Vater. Courvoisier's sign (a palpable enlarged gallbladder) occurs in only about 30% of patients. Pruritis is, of course, common and may tend to involve the palms and soles particularly. An epigastric mass is palpable in only about 20% of cases.

Symptomatic diabetes may have been recently diagnosed or may evolve after the diagnosis of cancer, but it is usually not very difficult to manage.

Trousseau's syndrome of migratory, often superficial, thrombophlebitis (named for both the patient and the physician, since Professor

Trousseau's self-diagnosis was confirmed at his autopsy) may also involve arterial thromboses and marantic endocarditis, but it is not really
very common.

Psychiatric problems ranging from mild personality change to severe
agitated depression to dementia are rather frequently seen. These have
frequently been noted to antedate the diagnosis of cancer by many
months or years, but chronic pain (which also often antedates diagnosis), failure of physicians to find a source of pain, disbelief by physicians and family of the seriousness of the symptoms, and other factors obviously must play significant roles in predisposing for emotional
and psychiatric disturbances.

Finally, pancreatic carcinoma often presents with liver, bone, lung,
or other metastases. In fact, it is the number one source of metastatic
adenocarcinoma when the primary is inapparent or unknown. Obviously, tumors arising in the body and tail are more prone to present
this way.


**Diagnosis**

Unfortunately, the *upper gastrointestinal series,* either with or without
hypotonic duodenography, is mainly sensitive to lesions that are both
large and involve the head of the gland. Besides a widened C-loop,
invasion of the posterior gastric wall and enlargement of the retrogas-
tric space may be seen.

The *pancreatic scan* turns out to be a procedure of little usefulness
(27). There are numerous false positives, but it has been said that a
normal scan is relatively reassuring. Not so. The author has seen several pancreatic carcinomas with unequivocally normal scans.

*Ultrasound* may suggest a lesion but does not reliably distinguish
between pancreatitis and tumor. Transhepatic cholangiography is only
used when the patient is ready to be taken immediately to surgery
should biliary sepsis ensue.

The place of the abdominal *computerized tomography* has yet to be
determined. So far this noninvasive technique has successfully identified large and/or already documented tumors in the pancreas, but it
has not been very reliable with smaller lesions.

The two most reliable diagnostic tests are both somewhat invasive.
Selective or superselective *arteriography* with various modifications

yields 85–95% accuracy with arterial obstruction, narrowing or encasement being common diagnostic findings. In addition to its diagnostic usefulness, angiography may provide valuable information regarding potential resectability.

*Endoscopic retrograde cholangiopancreatography* (ERCP) is a newer technique and still not widely available except in large centers (11,12). However, a similarly high accuracy (perhaps 90%) is claimed. Pancreatic ductal stenosis, occlusion, encasement or deformity, and necrotic cavity formation are the usual diagnostic signs. This technique is now being combined with CEA determinations, cytology, and/or bicarbonate levels after secretin testing to improve the overall results.

*Carcinoembryonic antigen* level is elevated in the majority of patients and very high levels (>10–20) tend to point particularly to the colon or pancreas. However, "early" pancreatic carcinoma has lower levels, and these may also be seen with benign pancreatic disease as well as numerous other conditions (see discussion under "Colorectal Carcinoma.")

A rather specific oncofetal antigen was described in 1974 (18), and considerable work is being done to confirm this and develop a clinically useful test.

Finally, it should be mentioned that, although *biopsy* of the pancreas has been a surgical anathema for years, recent series have demonstrated that either wedge or needle biopsy at exploratory laparotomy was well tolerated (total complication rate = 6.2%, no deaths) (17). In fact, needle biopsy under peritoneoscopic or ultrasonic guidance is now being investigated.

**Treatment**

*Surgical* Only 10% or so of patients will be found to be candidates for potentially curative surgery by total pancreatectomy or Whipple's procedure. The major morbidity of these operations is 50% and the mortality 10–40%. Despite this, no more than 2–20% survive 5 years (13,15). With the operative mortality higher than the cure rate, extremely careful selection is obviously in order.

On the other hand, biliary diversion by cholecysto- or choledochojejunostomy and a Bilroth II gastrojejunostomy provide important symptomatic relief for the majority of patients with unresectable pancreatic carcinoma and actually increased survival slightly in some series.

*Radiation and Chemotherapy*   For patients whose unresectable cancer is confined to the region of the pancreatic bed and immediately adjacent structures, the combined use of a split course of radiation to the pancreatic region plus 5-FU chemotherapy has been shown to increase survival. In one series, Moertel (16) randomized patients to radiation and placebo versus radiation + 5-FU. The mean survivals were 6.3 months versus 10.4 months, respectively.

The GI Tumor Study Group tested 6000 rads alone, versus 6000 rads + 5-FU, versus 4000 rads + 5-FU, using split-course radiation in all instances. 5-Fluorouracil was continued indefinitely after radiation was completed. The 1-year survivals were 13%, 36%, and 45% and the median survivals were 17, 35, and 46 weeks, respectively. More patients have subsequently been entered in the radiation + 5-FU arms to sort out any possible difference, but the combination of the two modalities seems superior to either alone.

*Chemotherapy Alone*   For more advanced disease, chemotherapy is of minimal effectiveness (14). 5-Fluorouracil gives about 20% objective responses for 2–4 months. Several series have claimed superiority (response rate ca. 30%) for the combination of 5-FU + BCNU. Newer combinations are being tested, the most promising of which at this time is Streptozotocin (an investigational drug) + Mitomycin-C + 5-FU. However, no regimen presently available seems to be more than marginally or occasionally effective, and none should be considered standard. It is recommended that patients be entered into therapeutic protocols when it is convenient for them, since the overall outlook remains so dismal for the individual patient.

*Other Therapeutic Measures*   The future directions of research include the development of new chemotherapeutic agents and radiation sensitizers and the use of fast neutrons, which do not require tissue oxygenation and have a greater biologic effectiveness, for radiation.

Attempts to improve pain control are increasingly taking place, and percutaneous splanchnic block is often useful. In our experience Methadone provides better analgesia with less habituation, sedation, and constipation (and at a lower price to the patient) than other narcotics. The Brompton's solution (heroin or morphine plus cocaine) is another alternative for control of pain in a terminal patient.

## GASTRIC ADENOCARCINOMA

### General Considerations

It is well known that the incidence of gastric cancer has spontaneously decreased in the U.S. to about 1/3 of its rate earlier in the century. This remains completely unexplained but, on a worldwide basis, gastric cancer tends to be less frequent wherever colon cancer is common and the U.S. incidence of the latter is rising. In any case, 14,000 gastric cancer deaths occur in the U.S. annually, about 5% of cancer deaths overall. In Japan, Chile, Iceland, and Finland the incidence is much higher. Japanese immigrating to the U.S. experience a reduction in risk the longer they live here, strongly suggesting an environmental influence.

Males are affected more often than females, and the peak incidence is at about age 55.

Various peculiarities of regional diets have been proposed as etiologic factors, but none has been very persuasively demonstrated. The increasing use of antioxidant preservatives in foods in the U.S. has been suggested as a cause of the declining rate here.

The only *demonstrated* risk factors are: (1) *gastric polyps*, which are possibly precancerous, and (2) various conditions in which *hypochlorhydria* is the common element: (a) *chronic atrophic gastritis* (which is, however, quite common in the older age groups), (b) *achlorhydria*, and (c) *previous gastric surgery* for peptic ulcer disease. In *pernicious anemia*, 5–10% of patients develop gastric cancer, about 22 times the attack rate in the normal population. The disease tends to be multicentric in these patients (21).

### Pathology and Staging

Fifty percent of cases involve the pyloris and/or antrum and 18% the lesser curvature, accounting for the majority. Twenty-one percent arise in the body and 7%, in the cardia. Although only 2–3% are found along the greater curvature, gastric ulcers in this location are highly suspicious since benign ulcers of the greater curvature are even rarer.

There are four growth patterns: (1) ulcerating tumors (75% of gastric cancer), (2) polypoid cancers (occur in 10% and are somewhat more favorable than the average), (3) scirrhous tumors (10% average; more, in nonsurgical series), thickening and stiffening the stomach either locally or diffusely as linitis plastica, and (4) superficial spreading tumors (in 5%; usually surgically curable) (20). For all types, the survival with unresectable disease is proportional to the degree of differentiation.

Variables important in staging are depth of invasion of bowel wall, involvement of perigastric lymph nodes on one or both curvatures, and presence of distant metastases.

|  | STAGE | 2-YEAR SURVIVAL | 5-YEAR SURVIVAL |
|---|---|---|---|
| IA | Confined to mucosa—negative nodes | 98% | 88% |
| IB | As far as serosa | | |
| IC | Penetration of serosa with or without contiguous invasion | 80% | 55% |
| II | Linitis plastica type *or* involved nodes on one side only | 47% | 25% |
| III | Nodes on both sides or at a distance | 30% | 10% |
| IV | Distant metastases | <10% | <5% |

Gastric tumors may spread by direct extension to involve the greater and lesser omenta, transverse colon or mesocolon, spleen or gastrosplenic ligament, pancreas, diaphragm, superior meresteric or celiac vessels, liver, abdominal wall, and possibly the left adrenal gland and kidney.

Rich lymphatic plexi are present in the submucosal and subserosal layers. The former communicates with its counterpart in the esophagus and the latter with a similar plexus in the duodenum, accounting for frequent spread to those structures. In fact, the lymphatic drainage of the stomach is so rich that a complete node dissection may not be feasible in principle. Besides the primary drainage to the gastric and gastroepiploic chains (lesser and greater curvatures), secondary drainage to the entire celiac axis (porta hepatis, splenic–suprapancreatic, retropancreaticoduodenal areas) and to the para-aortic nodes may occur. Further lymphatic drainage is to the left supraclavicular and axillary nodes.

Hematogenous spread is to the liver (ca. 30% of operated patients), lungs, bones, brain, and abdominal wall.

Peritoneal involvement is common, but may be limited to a single area, at least for awhile. In a series of patients undergoing "second-look" operations, some type of local or regional failure had occurred in 54%, distant spread in 30% (Gunderman and Sosin). Nearly half of the peritoneal disease was localized. Such findings may bear on strategies for adjuvant therapy.

**Diagnosis**

*Symptoms and Signs*  Vague abdominal discomfort, sometimes even in the lower abdomen, is the most common, and usually the first, problem. By the time this progresses to frank pain, the tumor may be unresectable. Anorexia, weight loss, early satiety, nausea, and vomiting are common also and occur earlier with pyloric lesions. Symptoms of anemia are also frequent.

An abdominal mass is usually an ominous sign of unresectable cancer. Other signs of distant spread include Virchow's (left supraclavicular) and Irish's (left anterior axillary) nodes, Blumer's shelf (rectal implants), Krukenberg tumors (ovarian metastasis), and the Sister Mary Joseph sign (periumbilical subcutaneous metastasis). Remote effects of gastric or other internal cancer include dermatomyositis and *Acanthosis nigricans.*

*Workup*  A careful upper GI series is quite accurate in establishing a diagnosis, *except* for small prepyloric lesions, for lesions of the cardia that have not obstructed, and occasionally for equivocal gastric ulcers (22). All three problems can be difficult for the gastroscopist to sort out as well. First, the cardia is the most difficult area to visualize, even with the fiberscope. Second, the appearance of an ulcer may be equivocal under direct vision as well as on upper GI series. Third, gastroscopic biopsies are tiny superficial bites, and the cancer may be largely submucosal. Therefore, a negative biopsy by no means rules out gastric cancer.

When the findings are equivocal, the detection of gastric achlorhydria will strongly suggest malignancy in a patient with an ulcer. Exfoliative cytology collected by the endoscopist may establish the diagnosis. A CEA above 5 would also be very suspicious. Finally, a repeat upper GI series in 4 weeks should demonstrate healing; a "benign-looking" ulcer that does not heal significantly in that period warrants an exploration (22). It should be recalled that the surgical approach to gastric ulcer disease, even if it proves benign, is highly satisfactory and has some advantages considering the high relapse rate of benign gastric ulcers.

Preoperative workup should include careful examination of the areas mentioned above (see "Symptoms and signs" section), roentgenograms of the entire GI tract, CEA, chest x-ray, and liver scan to rule out metastases *before* extensive surgery.

### Therapy and Prognosis

*Surgery*   Seventy-five to ninety percent of patients are found to be eligible for laparotomy and 50–60%, for potentially curative resection.

For cardia and proximal lesions, a total gastrectomy is preferred by most surgeons to avoid leakage of an esophageal–gastric anastomosis. For distal lesions, adequate en bloc subtotal gastrectomy is performed. Regional lymph-node dissection and resection, as necessary, of involved adjacent organs is carried out, even including the transverse colon or a portion of the liver, except that extension into the head of the pancreas is usually felt to be inoperable. A Bilroth II anastomosis is preferable to lessen the chance of outlet obstruction if there is a recurrence of tumor.

Unfortunately, only 15–20% of patients are Stage I, but 55–60% of these are cured. For the remainder, the 5-year survival is 7–12% (see previous breakdown by stage in "Pathology" section).

There is evidence that palliative resection or bypass in the incurable patient yields a longer survival, but in the patient known to be incurable before operation such a potential benefit has to be weighed against the extent of disease, operative risk, and other factors. The median survival with or without such therapy, ranges from 4–12 months.

*Radiation Therapy*   Although radiation alone does not seem to have much role except for symptomatic treatment of bony metastases, the combination of 5-FU + radiation in a controlled study of unresectable disease was superior to radiation alone in that the *mean* survival was prolonged by 6–14 months. However, the *median* survival was just barely prolonged, so that the effect of combined therapy was only apparent in a minority of patients (16). A study by Falkson also suggested an advantage to combined therapy over either modality alone. However, the development of better chemotherapy, described next, has possibly altered the apparent advantage to chemotherapy plus radiation.

*Chemotherapy*   For years, gastric tumors were poorly responsive to chemotherapy, felt to be even less responsive than colon cancer to 5-FU. Not only was that not true (there is the same 20–30% objective response to 5-FU), but several other active agents have since been identified: BCNU, Methyl-CCNU, Mitomycin-C, and Adriamycin.

Several combinations of these drugs have been established, the most promising of which are:

5-FU + BCNU
5-FU + Methyl-CCNU ± Vincristine
5-FU + Adriamycin + Mitomycin-C (FAM)

These all seem to give 40–55% objective tumor regression of advanced disease. These regressions are rarely complete, but FAM, for example, yielded 16 partial regressions (>50%) out of 29 patients, with a median duration of response of 9 months and median survival of the responders of over 12 months, compared to 2.5 months for the nonresponders. Such a respectable degree of activity for combination chemotherapy suggests that surgical adjuvant chemotherapy of resected gastric cancer may yet improve overall survival of this disease, and studies of this are now under way.

The superiority of simple 5-FU + radiation for the control of unresectable tumors has been mentioned above. Since the advent of combinations, this study has been repeated on a large scale by the Gastrointestinal Tumor Study Group, utilizing 5000 R + 5-FU (switching to Methyl-CCNU + 5-FU on completion of the radiation) and comparing to Methyl-CCNU + 5-FU from the outset without any radiation. Somewhat surprisingly, the preliminary analysis has shown a survival advantage for the combination chemotherapy-only group. Conceivably, the early utilization of effective chemotherapy has outweighed the benefit of a second modality of treatment.

*Supportive Therapy*   Adequate nutrition during therapy is apparently of great importance in increasing chances for effective palliation and in decreasing toxicity of radiation or chemotherapy. Where obstruction of the esophagus is present (in esophageal or gastric carcinoma), peroral nonoperative placement of an indwelling tube has proven surprisingly safe and offers excellent palliation (24,25). In less advanced cases, esophageal dilatation can be performed, and many patients can maintain patency by daily self-dilatation at home.

If oral intake cannot be maintained, intravenous hyperalimentation may be used to assure adequate nutrition during a course of therapy aimed at ultimately relieving the obstruction. Most oncologists tend to avoid placement of external enterostomies since these rarely are required except in the face of hopeless disease and under such circumstances are perhaps best withheld.

## REFERENCES

1. Proceedings of the Second National Conference on Cancer of the Colon and Rectum. Cancer 34: 799, 1974.
2. Proceedings of the Second Workshop on Large Bowel Cancer. Cancer 36: 2307, 1975.
3. Schein PS, Wooley PV III, Eds.: Colon carcinoma. Semin Oncol 3: 329, 1976.
4. Moertel CG, Reitemeier RJ: Advanced Gastrointestinal Cancer. Hoeber, New York, 1969.
5. Grage TB: Adjuvant chemotherapy with 5-fluorouracil after surgical resection of colorectal carcinoma. Am J Surg 133: 59, 1977.
6. Higgins GA: Adjuvant chemotherapy in surgical treatment of large bowel cancer. Cancer 38: 1461, 1976.
7. Moertel CG: Therapy of advanced colorectal cancer with a combination of 5-FU, methyl-CCNU and Vincristine. J Nat Cancer Inst 54: 69, 1975.
8. MacDonald JS: Current diagnosis and management of pancreatic carcinoma. J Nat Cancer Inst 56: 1093, 1976.
9. Krementz ET, Becker ML: Malignant diseases of the pancreas. Adv Surg 6: 205, 1972.
10. Cohn I: Cancer of the pancreas: Detection and diagnosis. Cancer 37: 582, 1976.
11. Silvis SE: Diagnostic accuracy of ERCP in hepatic, biliary and pancreatic malignancy. Ann Intern Med 84: 438, 1976.
12. White TT, Silverstein FE: Operative endoscopic pancreatography in the diagnosis of pancreatic cancer. Cancer 37: 449, 1976.
13. Brooks JR, Culebras JM: Cancer of the pancreas. Palliative operation, Whipple procedure or total pancreatectomy? Am J Surg 131: 516, 1976.

14. Carter SK, Comis RL: The integration of chemotherapy into a combined modality approach for cancer treatment. VI. Pancreatic adenocarcinoma. Cancer Treat Rev 2: 193, 1975.
15. Tepper J: Carcinoma of the pancreas: Review of MGH experience from 1963 to 1973. Analysis of surgical failure and implications for radiation therapy. Cancer 37: 1519, 1976.
16. Moertel CG: Combined 5-FU and supervoltage radiation therapy of locally unresectable gastrointestinal cancer. Lancet 2: 865, 1969.
17. Isaacson R: Biopsy of the pancreas. Arch Surg 109: 227, 1974.
18. Banwo O: New oncofetal antigen for human pancreas. Lancet 1: 643, 1974.
19. Moertel CG: Clinical management of advanced gastrointestinal cancer. Semin Drug Treat 3: 55, 1973.
20. Remine WH, Ed.: Cancer of the Stomach. Saunders, Philadelphia, 1964.
21. Huffman NR: The relationship between pernicious anemia and cancer of the stomach. Geriatrics 25: 90, 1970.
22. Larson NE: Prognosis of the medically treated small gastric ulcer: Comparison of follow-up data in two series. NEJM 264: 119, 1961.
23. Gunderson LL: Implications for adjuvant radiation therapy. Paper presented at Digestive Disease Week (postgraduate course of the American Gastroenterological Association), San Antonio, Texas, May 17–18, 1975.
24. Palmer ED: Peroral prosthesis for the management of incurable esophageal carcinoma. Am J Gastroenterol 59: 487, 1973.
25. Boyce HW Jr: Nonsurgical measures to relieve distress of late esophageal carcinoma. Geriatrics 28: 97, 1973.
26. Stern JL: Evaluation of palliative resection in advanced carcinoma of the stomach. Surgery 77: 291, 1975.
27. Barkin J et al: Computerized tomography, diagnostic ultrasound and radionuclide scanning: Comparison of efficacy in diagnosis of pancreatic carcinoma. JAMA 238: 2040, 1977.

# LUNG CANCER

OLEG S. SELAWRY, M.D., LAWRENCE E. BRODER, M.D.

## INCIDENCE

Lung cancer is the most commonly lethal cancer in the U.S. (and an increasing number of other countries), causing one of every three cancer deaths in males and one of every nine cancer deaths in females (Table 1). The incidence is 3–4 times greater in males than females. The incidence of lung cancer continues to rise faster than that of any other major cancer. This rate increase is steeper for women than for men.

**TABLE 1**

*Incidence of Lung Cancer in the U.S.: Estimates for 1977*

| | NUMBER OF PATIENTS | | |
| --- | --- | --- | --- |
| | DIAGNOSED | EXPIRED | CANCER DEATHS |
| All patients | 98,000 | 89,000 | 23% |
| Males | 76,000 | 68,300 | 33% |
| Females | 22,000 | 20,700 | 11% |

## ETIOLOGY

There is a strong relationship between cigarette smoking and lung cancer. "Ever-smokers" have 20–25 times more squamous-cell and small-cell cancer of the lung than "never-smokers." Lung cancer is also increased in uranium miners, coal-tar, chromate, nickel, arsenic (insecticides), paper, and asbestos workers (ship yards, auto mechanics, etc.) One or more of these agents are cocarcinogens (Table 2).

TABLE 2

*Lung Cancer in Four Risk Groups; Serial Follow-Up in 5765 Men*

| CYTOLOGY | URANIUM MINERS | | | |
| | SMOKERS | | NONSMOKERS | |
|---|---|---|---|---|
| Patient number | 1628 | 2496 | 1209 | 432 |
| Invasive carcinoma | | | | |
|   Epidermoid | 51 | 66 | 0 | 0 |
|   Small-cell | 8 | 81 | 1 | 0 |
| Total number, carcinomas | 59 | 147 | 1 | 0 |
| Total percent carcinomas | 3.6 | 5.9 | .08 | 0 |

*Data from Saccomanno et al., 1974.*

## MORPHOLOGIC CLASSIFICATION

Lung cancer encompasses several morphologically and clinically distinct disease entities. The classification of the World Health Organization as modified by Matthews and Yesner finds increasing acceptance and includes:

1. EPIDERMOID (SQUAMOUS-CELL) CARCINOMA. Approximately 50% of all lung cancer. Well differentiated, moderately well differentiated, poorly differentiated. The latter is frequently assigned to item 4 (below).
2. SMALL-CELL UNDIFFERENTIATED CARCINOMA. Approximately 15% of all lung cancers.
   a. Oat-celled (or lymphocyte-like).
   b. Other.
3. ADENOCARCINOMA. Approximately 15% of all lungs cancer. Well differentiated, moderately differentiated, poorly differentiated (see also item 4). Bronchioloalveolar (or papillary adeno-) carcinoma is an important subtype which is characterized by endobronchial extension.
4. LARGE-AND GIANT-CELL CARCINOMA is a particularly malignant subtype. Approximately 15% of all lung cancer.

5. Mixed types of carcinoma, including epidermoid and adenoma-tous cell elements.

6. Less common types of lung cancer such as sarcoma, mesothe-lioma, carcinoid, melanocarcinoma, etc. (less than 4% of all lung cancers).


## STAGING

The staging of the American Joint Committee is based on clinical find-ings; these may be refined by postsurgical staging.

T = Primary tumor.

TO— No evidence of primary tumor.

TX— Cytologic proof of tumor but no visualization on chest films or bronchoscopy.

T1— Greatest diameter up to 3 cm surrounded by lung or visceral pleura and without evidence of invasion proxi-mal to the lobar bronchus at bronchoscopy.

T2— Greatest diameter exceeds 3 cm or a tumor of any size, extending to the hilar region. The proximal tumor mar-gin must be at least 2 cm from the carina. Any associated atelectasis or obstructive pneumonitis must involve less than an entire lung, and there must be no pleural effu-sion.

T3— Tumors exceeding the above dimensions.

N = Regional lymph nodes.

N0— No demonstrable tumors in the regional nodes.

N1— Ipsilateral hilar involvement (including direct exten-sion).

N2— Mediastinal lymph nodes involved.

M = Metastases beyond N2.

M0 — No evidence for distant metastases.

M1— Distant metastases.

NOTE: The system can be expanded by designations such as:

M1.10 — Ipsilateral scalene and cervical lymph nodes involved.

M1.11 — Contralateral scalene and cervical lymph nodes involved.
M1.12 — Ipsilateral pleural effusion, etc.

T, N, and M are grouped into stages:

Stage 0 = Occult carcinoma, TX, NO, MO with positive cytology.
Stage 1 = Either of the following: T1, N0, M0, 5 year survival 40%
                                    T1, N1, M0
                                    T2, N0, M0
Stage 2 = T2, N1, M0.
Stage 3 = More extensive tumors.

Survival depends on both stage and cell type, epidermoid carcinoma showing the best survival and small-cell carcinoma showing the worst, because epidermoid carcinoma remains regional (devoid of distant, hematologic metastases) until death in approximately 50% of all patients, while small-cell carcinoma is associated with very early lymphogenous and hematogenous spread with distant metastases in 95% of patients at the time of death. Adeno- and large-cell carcinoma take an intermediate position.


## PRESENTATION

The onset is often insidious, with increased tiredness and some weight loss as systemic manifestations. The following signs and symptoms are pathognomonic:

1. Local disease present with increased cough with or without sputum, with or without hemoptysis.
2. Regional extension might manifest itself in hoarseness, Horner's syndrome (mediastinal extension), chest pain with or without extension to the bronchial plexus (pleural involvement; extension to the chest wall), or superior vena caval obstruction.
3. Metastatic disease might provide the presenting symptoms and signs of cerebral metastases, hepatic metastases, or osseous metastases.
4. Osteoarthropathy with clubbing of the fingers and toes occurs in some 10–20% of all patients with lung cancer.

5. Endocrine markers occurs in all cell types and might be associated with hypercalcemia in the absence of osseous metastases (epidermoid carcinoma), gynecomastia, Cushing's syndrome, or inappropriate ADH secretion.
6. Nonendocrine markers such as CEA (carcinoembryonic antigen) are noted in patients with all cell types of lung cancer and are useful for follow-up if the initial values exceed 5 mg/ml.

Changes listed under items 3–6 might precede the symptoms and signs of locoregional disease.


## WORKUP

Microscopic verification of the diagnosis by cell type is the key to therapy and should be attempted as soon as possible. The following techniques are employed.


### Sputum Cytology

This procedure can be used for cases described in items 3–5 (above) who present with deep cough, early-morning sputa, which may be aided by steam inhalation, if necessary. Sputum cytology should be diagnostic in some 80% of all patients with epidermoid carcinoma and with bronchioloalveolar carcinoma, while lower figures apply to the other cell types. The yield also increases with more central location of the tumor.


### Bronchoscopy

Bronchoscopy is desirable for diagnosis (bronchial brushings, biopsy), estimation of endobronchial extent and follow-up.


### Mediastinoscopy

Some lung cancers present as mediastinal tumors, and others show up as hilar masses. Mediastinoscopy often gives positive results and helps determine resectability. Seventy-five percent of lung-cancer patients have positive mediastinal nodes, foremost small-cell carcinoma, and least frequently well or moderately well-differentiated epidermoid carcinoma.

### Scalene Node Biopsy

Positive results are obtained when nodes are palpable. The right lung drains to the right nodes plus the left lower lobe. The left nodes drain the lingula and left upper lobe.

### Metastatic Workup

This includes brain scan, bone scan, and bone-marrow aspirate plus needle biopsy if the scan is equivocal, with no clear-cut evidence of metastatic disease. Small-cell carcinoma has tumor cells in 20–40% of marrow aspirates and biopsies; corresponding figures for adeno- and large-cell carcinoma are 10–20%. The incidence for epidermoid carcinoma stays below 10%. Liver metastases are common. They occur in 8–25% of otherwise resectable patients (depending on cell type) and in 30–60% of patients at autopsy. Increased alkaline phosphastase LDH and SGOT and liver scans might require confirmation by laparoscopy when the liver is the only site of suspected metastatic spread.

## COURSE AND PROGNOSIS

The following patterns are significant.

### Primary Site and Spread

Most cancers originate from segmental or subsegmental bronchi and spread rapidly endobronchially toward the hilar and mediastinal lymph nodes. Adenocarcinoma might invade the pulmonary parenchyma before spreading elsewhere; it has the highest incidence of pleural effusion. Bronchioloalveolar carcinoma shows the most extensive endobronchial spread. Small-cell carcinoma has the most extensive hilar and mediastinal involvement, with rapid spread to supraclavicular and subdiaphragmatic lymph nodes and to distant sites.

## Growth Speed

Average volume doubling times of well-outlined lung lesions are 1 month for small-cell carcinoma, 3–4 months for epidermoid and large-cell carcinoma, and 6 months for adenocarcinoma.

## Prognosis

The following guidelines might be of help.

*Local Disease, Resectable; 5-Year Survival*   For Stage 1, the 5-year survival rate is 35–40%; for groups T1, N0, and M0 it is 40–50%. For Stage 2, the rate is 10–15% and for Stage 3, less than 10%. Exceptions are as follows: (1) for small-cell carcinoma, groups T1, N0, and M0 with asymptomatic peripheral nodules, the rate is 35–40%; (2) all other resectable diseases are less than 5%. For superior-sulcus/pancoast tumor (Stage 3) with preoperative radiotherapy the rate is 20–40%.

*Regional Disease, Unresectable; 5-Year Survival with Intensive Radiotherapy*   The median survival rate is 4–10%. The rate for untreated cases is 4–6 months, shortest for small-cell and longest for epidermoid carcinomas.

*Extensive Disease with Metastases Beyond One Hemithorax and Corresponding Supraclavicular Nodes*   There is virtually no 5-year survival rate. Median survival is 1.5–4 months, shortest for small-cell and longest for epidermoid carcinomas. Modifying factors are ambulation, weight loss, delayed hypersensitivity tests (*Candida,* Mumps), and DNCB.

## TREATMENTS OF CHOICE

### Local Disease, Resectable and Operable:

*Surgery*   This is the treatment of choice. For 5-year survival rates, see under "Prognosis" section, "Local disease, resectable." Surgical lethality is 5–12%, depending on extent of procedure, age, and general condition of the patient. However, there is one exception; radiotherapy is at least as "good," probably better for 5-year survival of patients with resectable small-cell carcinoma other than the asymptomatic coin lesion.

*Surgery Plus Other Modalities:* Presurgical radiotherapy is of benefit for superior sulcus tumors. In all other situations there is no proof for improved survival following pre- or postsurgical radiotherapy. Surgical adjuvant chemotherapy has no established place, with the possible exception of small-cell carcinoma. Surgical adjuvant immunotherapy is experimental at this time. Intrapleural instillation of BCG is under investigation, as is the use of tumor-associated antigens. Levamisole might be of benefit for patients with Stage 2–3 epidermoid carcinoma.

### Regional, Unresectable Disease

*Radiotherapy* This modality offers 5-year survival in approximately 4–10% of patients with small lesions. Tumor shrinkage of 50% or better of well-outlined lesions is afforded in 60–70% of patients with small-cell carcinoma and in 30–50% of patients with other cell types. The majority of patients notice symptomatic improvement. Survival gains occur especially in patients with epidermoid carcinoma.

The following special cases are noted. For superior vena cava obstruction, radiotherapy is the treatment of choice. For cerebral metastases, corticosteroids are as effective as radiotherapy for short-term control (weeks). Radiotherapy of the whole brain to the equivalent of 5000 rads in 5 weeks is usually sufficient for long-term palliation.

*Combination of Radiotherapy Plus Chemotherapy* Combination of these two modalities might be beneficial for small-cell carcinoma. For all other cell types, the data are controversial. Combination of radiotherapy with nonspecific immunostimulation might be of benefit (BCG in one prospective, controlled clinical trial).

*Chemotherapy Alone or Plus Radiotherapy* Chemotherapy followed by radiotherapy or chemotherapy alone is the treatment of choice for small-cell carcinoma, with tumor regression in 60–90% of the patients, complete tumor regression in 20–50+% of the patients, and median survival of 12+ months in the best recent studies.

### Metastatic Disease or Regional Progressive Disease after Radiotherapy

The indications for treatment and the choice of drugs depends on the cell type.

*Epidermoid Carcinoma* Tumor shrinkage of 50% or better occurs in 20–35% of the patients and is indicated for palliation of symptoms.

Single drugs are probably as effective as drug combinations, as judged by results of controlled clinical trials. Methotrexate twice weekly per-orally results in reasonable palliation; responders live 2–3 times longer than nonresponders. Nonresponders live as long as placebo-treated patients.

*Small-cell Anaplastic Carcinoma* Single drugs and drug combinations are more effective when used as early as possible. Drug combinations are more effective than the best single drugs, with response rates of 50–90% and median survivals of 8–14 months for the best current regimens. Examples for two non-cross-resistant combinations are as follows:

Adriamycin + Procarbazine + Vincristine
Cytoxan + CCNU + Methotrexate

Other combinations are similarly effective but make it difficult to reinduce response after relapse.

Other non-cross-resistant drugs or drug combinations might be used for control of disease after a second relapse.

*Adenocarcinoma* Combinations with response rates above 30% include Cytoxan + CCNU + Methotrexate, Cytoxan + Methotrexate to leukopenia of 2–3000 and 5-FU + Procarbazine. Vincristine, Mitomycin, Methorexate, and Cyclophosphamide are among the more effective single agents.

*Large-cell Carcinoma* Response rates approaching 40% occur with drug combinations that include Adriamycin (Adriamycin + Cytoxan + DTIC or Vincristine). Procarbazine, Cyclophosphamide, and Methyl-CCNU are among the more effective single drugs.

## REFERENCES

1. Selawry OS, Hansen HH: Lung cancer. pp 1473–1518, *In* Cancer Medicine, Ed. J. F. Holland and E. T. Frei, Lea & Febiger, Philadelphia, 1973 (2nd ed. 1978).
2. Israel L, Chahinian P, Ed.: Lung Cancer, Facts, Concepts and Strategies. Academic Press, New York, 1976.
3. Straus M, Ed.: Lung Cancer. Clinical Diagnosis and Treatment. Grune and Stratton, New York, San Francisco, London, 1977.

# GENITOURINARY CANCER

## NORMAN L. BLOCK, M.D.

### CANCER OF THE KIDNEY

**Epidemiology**

Renal cancer is the second most common urinary tract tumor in adults, accounting for approximately 1% of all cancers, with approximately 11,000 new cases each year. The age of diagnosis averages 55–60 years, and there is a 2:1 male predominance. In the past 30 years there has been an approximate doubling of the incidence rate of kidney cancer. During the same time span there has been a definite, but very slight, shift to earlier diagnosis. Approximately 80% of kidney tumors are adenocarcinomas or hypernephromas; 15% are transitional cell or squamous cell tumors of the renal pelvis, and 5% are sarcomas and other uncommon tumors (2).

**Etiology**

Adenocarcinomas of the kidney have been etiologically associated with smoking and several hormone abnormalities. A genetic predisposition is occasionally seen. Experimentally, tumors can be produced with an assortment of hormone preparations, and experimentally and epidemiologically there seems to be an association between kidney cancer and exposure to lead. Squamous- and transitional-cell tumors of the pelvis have been associated with chronic inflammation, renal stone disease, and phenacetin abuse (1).

**Clinical Symptoms and Diagnosis**

The most frequent symptoms associated with kidney cancer are hematuria, pain, flank mass, fever, and polycythemia. A wide range of nonspecific symptoms such as fatigue, weight loss, gastrointestinal symptoms and anemia, is also seen. In addition, such clinical problems as hypercalcemia, hepatopathy, polyneuritis, congestive heart failure, varicocele, hypertension, and an assortment of paraneoplastic syndromes can be seen.

A wide range of diagnostic procedures is available. Hematuria revealed on urinalysis may provide the first clue. Excretory urography may reveal a mass in the kidney, or a filling defect in the pelvis. Approximately 10–15% of renal tumors are discovered serendipitously on IVPs done for unrelated reasons. Retrograde pyelography may occasionally be of use in better delineating a kidney structure poorly visualized on IVP. Nephrotomography is useful in clarifying the presence or absence of a mass defect or irregularity of the renal outline, and is also helpful in differentiating cyst and solid mass. Selective renal angiography is extremely useful and shows characteristic neovasculature in 90–95% of tumors. Venacavography can occasionally be useful in demonstrating distortion and displacement of the vena cava, invasion of the cava by tumor, and the presence of tumor in the renal veins draining into the cava. Urinary cytology may be of some use in tumors of the renal pelvis; however, cytology is extremely undependable in adenocarcinomas. Ultrasonography may be useful in differentiating cystic from solid masses. Needle aspiration of cystic masses may provide fluid for cytologic and chemical testing and enable differentiation between necrotic cystic tumors and benign cysts. Thin-needle aspiration of known tumors may also provide useful cytologic material.

## Staging (1)

STAGE 1A: INTRARENAL, INTRACAPSULAR. The tumor is encapsulated and the capsule is intact without renal parenchymal invasion.

STAGE 1B: INTRARENAL, EXTRACAPSULAR. The tumor capsule is broken and the renal parenchyma is invaded, but there is no involvement of veins, lymphatics, or renal capsule.

STAGE 2: PERINEPHRIC, MICROSCOPIC. There is an invasion through the renal capsule into the perinephric fat and microscopic evidence of venous and lymphatic invasion. The gross disease is resectable with only microscopic residuum.

STAGE 3: PERINEPHRIC, GROSS. There is invasion into the perinephric fascia, gross lymph node, and renal vein. Resection is incomplete, and obvious gross disease is left behind.

STAGE 4: DISTANT METASTASES. Visceral metastases to bone, lung, brain, and other sites are present.

## Treatment

Radical nephrectomy is the only required treatment for Stages 1 and 2. Radical nephrectomy is the treatment of choice, and there is no definite evidence that further adjunct radiation or chemotherapy is of any value for Stage 3. Radical nephrectomy is also the means of definitive staging and the primary treatment. There is preliminary evidence that radiation therapy, either preoperatively or to the tumor bed postoperatively, is of some value in preventing recurrence. For Stage 4, palliative nephrectomy is of very limited applicability. Renal pelvic tumors are best treated by nephroureterectomy, including a cuff of bladder. Renal sarcomas are best treated by radical nephrectomy.

The use of chemotherapeutic agents for renal carcinoma has not been very rewarding, although some of the newer agents have shown promise in isolated cases. Progesterone and testosterone are of value in relatively small numbers of cases, particularly in males with pulmonary metastases.

## Prognosis

For Stages 1 and 2, the 5-year survival rate is 30–50%; for Stage 3, it is 10–15% and for Stage 4, 0–2%. For transitional-cell carcinomas, the survival statistics for analogous stages are similar. Squamous-cell tumors of the renal pelvis are extremely aggressive, and 5-year survivals are rarely seen (1).

## CARCINOMA OF THE PROSTATE

### Epidemiology

Cancer of the prostate has the highest incidence of any cancer in men over 50 and is the third leading cause of death of males from cancer in the U.S. Ten percent of the deaths in the U.S. result from carcinoma of the prostate. Microscopic lesions may be found at autopsy in 15–20% of men in the fifth decade of life, rising to as high as 90% in the ninth decade; only 10% of these become clinically significant. The disease is more common in American blacks than in Caucasians and less common in Orientals than in Caucasians. There seems to be an increased incidence of prostate cancer in men with early puberty, early coitus, and numerous sexual partners.

## Pathology

Carcinoma reportedly arises more frequently in the posterior lobe of the prostate. However, careful autopsy studies reveal that tumors may arise anywhere in the prostate, the incidence being wholly dependent on the bulk of any particular lobe. Prostate cancer is adenocarcinoma in 99% of cases, with the remaining 1% being distributed among squamous-cell tumors and various sarcomas.

## Etiology

Although there have been considerable attempts to implicate hormonal changes as an etiologic factor in prostate cancer, no definite evidence has been forthcoming. There is strong suggestive evidence that in the natural state androgens encourage the growth of the tumor. However, this has been inadequately studied in humans. Virus-like particles (C-particles) have been reported in prostate cancer tissue.

## Symptoms and Diagnosis

Early prostate cancer is generally completely asymptomatic and may be discovered either by the pathologist following surgery for clinically benign disease or by the examining finger during a routine physical examination. If it is associated with benign prostatic hypertrophy, it may also be associated with lower-tract urinary symptoms, though not productive thereof. Approximately 50% of nodules detected on physical examination are shown to be neoplastic, and the remainder are generally prostatic calculi or chronic inflammatory changes with induration. Diagnosis is generally made by needle biopsy through the rectum or the perineum for early cases, and either needle biopsy or transurethral biopsy for advanced-stage tumors. Approximately 5–10% of tumors are discovered incidentally during treatment for benign disease, 5–10% are discovered by routine physical examination as isolated nodules, 40% of newly diagnosed tumors are Stage C (see under "Staging" section, to follow), meaning local advanced disease, and 40–50% of new tumors are Stage D with metastatic lesions. Stage D carcinomas presenting with metastases may be associated with a primary lesion ranging from a large rock-hard bulky prostate to a lesion that is not clinically appreciated in the prostate. A typical metastatic lesion on bone survey is an osteoblastic change; however, 10% of cases show either pure lytic or mixed lytic plus blastic lesions. Bone scans are generally more sensitive in picking up early metastases than are bone surveys and may also be of use in differentiating nonneo-plastic blastic changes from metastases. Serum acid phosphatase is a useful diagnostic tool and of some limited use prognostically; however, the test is notoriously unreliable with both false positives and false negatives, and it is difficult to make reliable judgment based on single determinations. Bone-marrow acid phosphatase remains in the category of limited applicability.

### Staging (1)

STAGE A: The tumor is found during pathologic examination of prostate tissue removed for clinically benign disease.

STAGE B: The isolated nodule is usually found on routine physical examination and is normally asymptomatic.

STAGE C: The disease extends beyond the prostate or prostate capsule into seminal vesicles and/or periprostatic fat or bladder base. Lower urinary tract symptoms are generally present.

STAGE D: In this stage there are distant metastases. The acid phosphatase is generally elevated, and symptoms of lower-tract obstruction are frequently present.

### Treatment (3,4,5)

STAGE A: Well-differentiated tumors in males with less than 15 years projected life span are best left untreated and closely observed. In males with greater than 15 years' expected life span or higher-grade tumors, either radical prostatectomy or some alternate form of therapy may be of use.

STAGE B: Radical prostatectomy or radiation therapy, by either interstitial or external routes, are the methods of choice. Radical prostatectomy has the disadvantage of causing impotence in almost all cases and incontinence in 10–20% of cases.

STAGE C: Patients in this category are best treated by radiation therapy by either interstitial or external routes.

STAGE D: The carcinoma is best treated by either orchiectomy or estrogen at the dose level of 1 mg per day. There does not seem to be any advantage to estrogen–orchiectomy combined. The question of the usefulness of higher doses of estrogen is still clouded. Hypophysectomy and adrenalectomy are occasionally useful after the patient's tumor becomes estrogen-independent. Various androgens are in the stage of early clinical testing. External radiation or $P^{32}$ isotope treatment may be useful to relieve local bone pain or obstruction. An assortment of cytotoxic chemotherapeutic agents, both singly and combined, may produce objective responses in small numbers of cases.

### Prognosis (3)

The 5-year survival rate is 75% for Stage A, 60% for Stage B, 35–40% for Stage C, and 10–20% for Stage D.

## TESTICULAR CARCINOMA

### Epidemiology

The incidence rate of testicular tumors in the U.S. is two per 100,000 males, or 1% of all cancers in males. These tumors account for 10–15% of all cancer deaths in the 15–34-year-old age group. Testicular tumors are uncommon in blacks, being about 10% of the incidence in Caucasians; the peak age in Caucasians for testicular tumor is 32. However, tumors may be seen in young males, where the most frequent tumor is embryonal carcinoma and in elderly males, where it is seminoma (1,6).

## Etiology

The chances of tumor development in an undescended testes is 10–80 times greater than a normal testes. Eleven percent of patients with testicular tumors give a history of trauma; however, despite a great deal of investigation, it is difficult to implicate this as an etiologic factor. In most cases, it seems that the trauma has called attention to the abnormal testicle rather than caused the tumor itself. Many patients with testicular tumors give a antecedent history of swelling of the testicle, which is followed for several weeks to several months with a tentative diagnosis of orchitis or epididymitis. There are a few cases of testicular tumors in brothers and father–sons; however, there does not seem to be a significant familial predilection.

## Pathology

Of testicular tumors, seminoma comprises 35–40%, embryonal carcinoma 15–20%, and teratoma and teratocarcinoma 20–30%, and some combination of the above is seen in 15–40% of tumors. Pure choriocarcinoma comprises approximately 1% of testicular tumors.

## Staging (6)

STAGE 1A. The tumor is confined to one testes, and there is no clinical or radiographic evidence of spread beyond the testes.

STAGE B: Patients in this category exhibit the same findings as those in Stage 1A but show histologic evidence of metastases to iliac or paraortic lymph nodes at the time of lymphadenectomy.

STAGE 2. There is clinical or radiographic evidence of metastases to femoral, inguinal, or iliac or paraortic lymph nodes. There is no demonstrable metastases above the diaphragm or to visceral organs.

STAGE 3. There is clinical or radiographic evidence of metastases above the diaphragm or other distant metastases to body organs.

## Clinical and Diagnostic Findings

A painful swelling of the testes is the most common symptom, occurring in 65% of cases. Other symptoms include pain, 9% mass plus pain,

9% trauma, and 5% metastases. Metastases may be seen in the lungs, mediastinal nodes, brain, and supraclavicular nodes, the last sometimes occurring quite early in the course of the disease. Endocrine disturbances occur in about 5% of testicular tumors and in a very high percentage of choriocarcinomas. Human chorionic gonadatrophin $\alpha$-Fetoprotein is elevated in nonseminomatous testicular tumors and are extremely useful for following the progress of the disease (7).

## Therapy

The proper diagnostic and therapeutic procedure is high inguinal orchiectomy with clamping of the cord during exploration of the testicle if that is considered to be necessary. Needle biopsy and exploration through the scrotum are definitely contraindicated. Seminomas are extremely radiosensitive, and treatment may be limited to radiation only. The proper treatment for nonseminomatous testicular tumors is still not established. Retroperitoneal lymphadenectomy without radiation therapy, radiation therapy alone, and several "sandwich techniques" have all been advocated. A wide range of cytoxic chemotherapeutic agents has been applied with varying results for testicular tumors. These have included Vincristine, Actinomycin-D, Cytoxan, Bleomycin, Methotrexate, 5-FU, Velban, Adriamycin, and Mithramycin. Recently a combination of Velban, Bleomycin, and cis-platinum has produced extremely high response rates with prolonged remissions in many centers (1,6,8).

## Prognosis

The 5-year survival rates for Stages 1–3 are tabulated as follows (1).

|  | STAGE 1 | STAGE 2 | STAGE 3 |
|---|---|---|---|
| Seminoma | 98% | 34–76% | 7% |
| Embryonal | 74% | 3–36% | 8% |
| Teratocarcinoma | 78% | 7–47% | 0% |
| Choriocarcinoma | 100% | 0% | 0% |
| Mixed | 66–100% | 0–40% | 0–13% |

# BLADDER CANCER

## Epidemiology

Bladder cancer is the most frequent malignant tumor of the urinary tract. There is approximately a 3:1 male predominance, and 20,000 new cases of bladder cancer expected this year. Bladder cancer is the 11th highest cause of cancer deaths in the U.S. Over the past 30 years there has been a definite and significant trend toward earlier diagnosis and treatment.

## Etiology

Aniline dye used in rubber in cable industries is related to the induction of bladder cancer. Naphthylamine, Adminodiphenyl, and tobacco tar can cause bladder tumors in animals. Cigarette smoking may play a role in the human tumor. Chronic bladder infections and calculi as well as schistosomiasis are factors in development of squamous-cell carcinoma. Persons living in urban areas have a higher incidence of bladder cancer than those living in rural areas. There seems to be an increased frequency among workers in factories as opposed to white collar workers. Urinary bladder tumors are seen more frequently in single persons or those currently unmarried. A strong familiar link for bladder cancer has been observed. Bladder cancer shows its highest incidence in the northeastern U.S.

## Pathology

Eighty percent of tumors of the bladder are transitional-cell carcinoma, 15% are squamous-cell, and 5% are an assortment of uncommon carcinomas and sarcomas.

## Stage and Anatomic Staging

The system of Jewett is that most widely used in the U.S. and delineates tumors as follows: Stage 0, confined to superficial mucosa; Stage

A, submucosal infiltration; Stage B1, muscle invasion; Stage B2, deep muscle invasion; Stage C, perivesical infiltration; Stage D, spread metastatic disease. Common metastatic sites are regional lymph nodes, liver, lung, and bones (1). The histologic appearance of the tumor may give some indication of the biological potential. Most high-grade lesions are seen as high-stage lesions. The histologic grading of the lesion is of great significance in therapeutic decisions.

## Clinical and Diagnostic Findings

Gross hematuria is the most common finding in the first sign of 75% of bladder-cancer cases. Bladder irritability with frequency and dysuria occurs in about 1/3 of cases and increases with later stages of the disease. Bleeding is characteristically intermittent and is a factor in the delay to diagnosis since the patient and physician may both defer workup.

Urinalysis is useful in showing either microscopic or gross hematuria. Occasionally, exfoliated tumor cells may be seen in a urine grossly examined for routine urinalysis. Excretory urography is useful for the determination of upper-tract tumors or obstruction and location of bladder filling defects. Urinary cytology is of use in screening patients at high risk because of industrial carcinogenic exposure or a past history of bladder tumor. It is generally not cost-effective for diagnosis of the initial lesion. Cytoscopy, of course, is diagnostic and should generally be performed with the patient under anesthesia, so that a careful bimanual examination can be done to stage the tumor. Other recommended procedures are biopsy to determine grade and depth of infiltration, chest x-ray, skeletal survey, and bone and liver scans. Various optional studies include cystography, pelvic arteriography, and lymphangiography.

## Treatment

The following eight factors must be taken into account in determining the proper treatment for a particular bladder tumor: (1) anatomic–histologic classification, (2) location of tumor, (3) general health of the patient, (4) associated genitourinary problems such as compromised renal function, (5) ability of the patient to tolerate and care for a urinary appliance, (6) history of tumor recurrence and tumor grade, (7) history of previous surgery or radiation therapy, and (8) training and expertise of the surgeon or radiation therapist.

Surgical treatment may include endoscopic resection and fulguration for superficial slowly recurring tumors of low grade and low stage. It is also useful for control of bleeding and for those patients who are poor operative risks or have advanced disease. Segmented bladder resection is reserved for discrete lesions far from the bladder neck or ureteral orifices. For more advanced tumors, total cystectomy is the surgical procedure of choice. Cystectomy requires urinary diversion, which is most commonly a ureteroileal–cutaneous anastomosis. Radiation may be useful for patients with infiltrative lesions who do not desire surgery or who are not good operative candidates. It is also useful for palliation. External radiation therapy is the method of choice, although some experience with interstitial implantation has been reported. Mortality from radical cystectomy and urinary diversion is 5–12%, and mortality from the side effects of radiation therapy is approximately 6%. Topical chemotherapy in the form of Thio-tepa instillation to the bladder is of some use in controlling tumors in approximately 2/3 of patients. Other topical chemotherapeutic agents have not been reliable. Systemic cytotoxic chemotherapy shows objective responses in 5–15% of patients, most of these responses being relatively short in nature.

**Prognosis (2)**

| STAGE | SUPERVOLTAGE RADIATION | TOTAL CYSTECTOMY |
|-------|------------------------|------------------|
| O,A,B, | 12–71% | 32–80% |
| B2,C | 7–28% | 8–36% |
| D | 0% | 0–12% |
| Total | 6–33% | 13–43% |

The large range in these 5-year survival figures is due to patient selection, surgical and radiation therapist aggressiveness, and associated medical diseases.

# REFERENCES

1. Proceedings of the National Conference on Urologic Cancer. Cancer 32: 1017, 1973.
2. Silverberg E: Urologic cancer, statistical and epidemiological information. American Cancer Society.
3. Bailer JC, Byar DP, VA Cooperative Urological Research Group: Estrogen treatment for cancer of the prostate; early results with three doses of diethylstilbesterol and placebo. Cancer 26: 257, 1970.
4. National Prostatic Cancer Work Shop. Cancer Chemother Rep 59: 1, 1975.
5. Bagshaw MA: Definitive radiotherapy and carcinoma of the prostate. JAMA 210: 326, 1969.
6. Twito DI, Kennedy BJ: Treatment of testicular cancer. Ann Rev Med 26: 235, 1975.
7. Scardino PT, Cox HD, Waldmann TA, McIntire KR, Mittenmeyer B, Javadpour N: The value of serum tumor markers in the staging and prognosis of germ cell tumors of the testis. J Urol 118: 994, 1977.
8. Earle JD, Bagshaw MA, Kaplan HS: Supervoltage radiation therapy of the testicular tumors. Amer J Roentgenol Rad Ther Nucl Med 117: 653, 1973.

# SOFT-TISSUE AND BONE SARCOMAS

## MICHAEL B. TRONER, M.D.

This group of tumors remains a rare but challenging clinical entity. Sarcomas account for less than 1% of solid tumors in adults and in the pediatric population and younger adults, for 6% of the total tumors. The recent reports of increased survival utilizing multimodality approaches in diseases with generally poor prognoses have made treatment of sarcomas rewarding and have made it imperative that physicians be familiar with the appropriate therapeutic approaches.

The etiology of sarcomas has been extensively evaluated. Many varieties of sarcomas have been induced in laboratory animals by chemical carcinogens as well as viruses. In humans, oncogenic type C RNA virus with characteristic morphology has been observed. A viral pathogenesis is strongly suspected in human sarcomas, with a tumor-specific antigen isolated from human tumors. Morton and Eilber (1) showed 100% of patients with various soft-tissue and bone sarcomas to have antibody to this antigen, while 67% of family members and 25% of normal donors were also proven to have these antibodies. The presence of antibodies to the common antigens of sarcomas in both family members and normal donors suggests an unrecognized infection in these groups. Further evidence of a possible viral carcinogenesis has been the use of cell-free extracts of human bone cancer to induce sarcomas in newborn hamsters. A significantly higher number of mesenchymal tumors such as osteosarcoma and fibrosarcomas has been produced in these animals as compared to controls.

In recent experiments (2) that further support a viral pathogenesis, humoral antibodies and delayed hypersensitivity to sarcoma antigens have again been shown to exist in household contacts as well as patients with osteosarcoma. In parallel laboratory studies the mothers of tumor-bearing newborn hamsters develop similar antibodies after their offspring have been infected with sarcoma tumor viruses.

Primary bone tumors are far less common than metastatic tumors to the bone. Bone tumors are almost never picked up by the fortuitous radiographic examination of the bones. Dahlin's (3) exceptional review of the referral population at the Mayo Clinic reveals the order in descending frequency of primary bone tumor as osteosarcomas, chondrosarcoma, Ewing's sarcoma, and fibrosarcoma. Osteosarcoma has a bimodal distribution with a peak in the seventh decade and an earlier peak in the second. Childhood osteosarcomas are localized to the long bones of the lower limbs with a peak incidence at a mean age of 12.5 years in females and 16 years in males. This shows a close coincidence with the maximum growth velocity for the adolescent growth spurt of 12 years in females and 14 years in males. Osteosarcoma in older patients has been associated with long-standing Paget's disease, chronic osteomyelitis, bone infarct, and following radiation therapy for benign or malignant diseases.

The pathological interpretation of primary bone tumors can be difficult. They are classified according to the most differentiated tissue produced by the lesion. Osteoid, for example, must be present for the diagnosis of osteosarcoma, cartilage for the diagnosis of chondrosarcoma, and so on. The type of biopsy is important. Incisional biopsy appears to be preferred as long as it includes an adequate amount of tumor and some adjacent normal tissue. Biopsy of the frequently encountered central necrosis is to be avoided. The delay of definitive treatment by the use of incisional biopsy does not appear to have any significant bearing on the patient's ultimate prognosis.

Frequently tumors of bone are so undifferentiated that their primary is undefinable. This becomes important when clinical decisions related to amputation versus preservation of limbs are contingent on accurate histopathology. Electron microscopy can reveal differential characteristics in the cytoplasm and extracellular products that are not visualized by light microscopy. For example, the identification of glycogen in cytoplasm is a confirmatory sign of Ewing's sarcoma. Frequently it is unseen on light microscopy, even when present on electron microscopy. The cross-striations of rhabdomyosarcoma are frequently absent on light microscopy of poorly differentiated tumors but are easily detectable by electron microscopy. Other areas where electron microscopy is helpful are neurotubules in neuroepithelial tumors, desmosomes, tonofibrils, and tight junctions of epidermal carcinomas and premelanosomes of malignant melanoma. Electron microscopy demands prompt fixation in specific fixatives and adequate sampling of material. It is currently indicated only when the diagnosis cannot be made by light microscopy.

In addition to electron microscopy increasing the accuracy of histological diagnosis, pathologists have identified a new group of sarcomas. This is the so-called malignant fibrous histiocytoma and is now felt to be one of the more common sarcomas. In the past these were identified as adult fibrosarcomas or fibroxanthosarcomas. These lesions are located below the deep fascia, frequently on extremities, but they can also be found in the retroperitoneum, bones, and occasionally in parenchymal organs. Local excision of a malignant fibrous histiocytoma is frequently followed by recurrence or metastasis to lymph nodes or lungs. Hopefully, the continued reclassification of sarcomas will serve to simplify the clinician's approach to patients rather than confuse it.

Most patients with bone tumor present with pain, occasional swelling, and/or pathological fractures. Common sites of involvement of bone tumors vary depending on the primary tumor. Osteosarcomas are generally confined to the long bones, vertebrae, and mandible. Only eight out of 620 osteosarcomas in Dahlin's (3) series were distal to the ankle and wrist. Chondrosarcoma has localizations, with the addition of the rib cage, similar to those of fibrosarcoma. Ewing's sarcoma, though confined to an adolescent or even younger population than osteosarcoma, has a more equal distribution of tumors to all major sites including long bone, pelvis, ribs, and vertebrae.

Radiographic evaluation is important for localization, but rarely can it yield a definitive diagnosis. The mottled calcifications of chondrosarcoma, the sunburst spiculation of osteosarcoma, or the onion-skin pattern are suggestive of histologic type, and benign tumor must be ruled out. Radiology plays an important role in the attempts to stage the degree of local and/or distant invasion and to evaluate the most appropriate biopsy site. Whole-lung tomograms or computerized tomography (which may be more sensitive) are also important to rule out occult metastatic disease. Arteriograms are almost routinely utilized to define the local extent of the tumor and invasion of major blood vessels. Gallium and bone scans have also been useful in attempting to define extent of disease. Gallium has a 95% accuracy rate in soft-tissue sarcoma. It is especially useful in the detection of intra-abdominal disease and monitoring its response to chemotherapy or radiation therapy.

Laboratory studies are of minimal value in the diagnosis of primary bone tumor. The presence of monoclonal proteins in urine or serum can readily identify myeloma. Serum acid phosphatase elevations suggest metastatic prostatic carcinoma. Elevated levels of alkaline phosphatase are found in osteosarcoma and can predate clinical recurrence.

The clinical course of osteosarcoma and most bone tumors has usually been straightforward, with biopsy, then radical surgical extirpation, and usually the rapid development of metastatis to lung and/or other bones. At 2 years approximately 20% of patients survived without evidence of disease, and the remaining 80% had succumbed to tumor. The treatment of Ewing's sarcoma appeared more futile with 5-year survivals less than 15%. As with osteosarcoma, this was clearly related to widespread metastasis and not to local recurrence of tumor.

Current treatment of osteosarcoma illustrates recent dramatic changes in survival patterns with the report of 50–60% 2-year survival. The difference has been early and aggressive use of adjuvant chemotherapy following radical extirpative surgery. In the initial study reported by Jaffe (4), Vincristine, Methotrexate (utilizing extremely high doses), accompanied by citrovorum factor (CF) rescue, were effective in keeping adolescent patients free of metastatic disease. Citrovorum factor is the synonym for folinic acid, which provides the active metabolite tetrahydrofolate (the rescue) that is routinely blocked by methotrexate. Similar results were reported by others utilizing (5) Adriamycin as a single agent. Recently Jaffe has added Adriamycin to their regiment of V-MTX-CF. An additional 22 patients have been treated, only six of whom have had relapses (6).

The toxicity of these regimens can be considerable. Monitoring of Methotrexate levels by radioimmunoassay is important to adjust the length of CF Rescue. Appropriate hydration and attention to renal function is important, as Methotrexate excretion can be delayed and toxicity increased. Although still performed in a limited number of specialized centers, the continued excellent results with acceptable toxicity would dictate that adjuvant chemotherapy be considered in all juvenile osteosarcomas.

Success with this chemotherapy has prompted the use of less aggressive surgery in combination with drug treatment to avoid the trauma of amputation. Chemotherapy when given initially has reduced the size of primary tumors and in some cases has completely resolved pulmonary metastases present at initial diagnosis. Surgery with the use of internal bone prostheses and vigorous rehabilitation has been used in six patients in Boston. Five are still without evidence of disease with 1–17 months of follow-up. Similarly, Rosen (7) has performed prosthetic bone replacement in 15 patients, only one whom had recurrence and died. Two of the 15 patients required amputation at a later date. Although subamputative surgery requires considerable effort, if results in other hands continue to remain as favorable (80% of patients have a viable extremity), this should rapidly replace amputation as the primary surgical treatment.

Chemotherapy of clinically obvious metastatic bone sarcomas has been less successful. There are clearly active drugs such as Adriamycin (40% response rate), Cyclophosphamide, Adriamycin and Methotrexate in combination (35–40% response rate), and Cyclophosphamide, Vincristine, Actinomycin-D, or DTIC (40% response rate). Jaffe and Frei (6) recently utilized a weekly regimen of Methotrexate with CF Rescue as opposed to the every-3-week regimen they had used in adjuvant therapy. They have reported an 82% response rate with nine out of 11 patients in complete or partial remission. Further documentation by other investigators of the efficacy of this regimen is expected.

Surgical resection of single or few pulmonary metastatic lesions is an accepted procedure. Whether these patients would have survived without surgery is difficult to ascertain, but untreated patients with pulmonary metastatis have only a 5% 3-year survival rate from time of *initial amputation*. Selection factors appear to be: (1) disease-free interval of 24 months, (2) a tumor doubling time of more than 40 days, (3) limited number of resectable pulmonary nodules, (4) primary lesion remaining under control, and (5) ability of patient to tolerate surgery. Utilizing these criteria, 5-year survivals of 28% and 26% (8) have been reported. Hopefully, the addition of chemotherapy to this regimen will further improve survival rates.

The role of radiation therapy in osteosarcoma, chondrosarcoma, and fibrosarcoma of the bone appears to be limited. The utilization of high-dose radiation to long-bone tumors and observation for subsequent pulmonary metastasis prior to amputation has ceased to be a viable clinical approach. Five-year survivals are certainly no better than with surgery alone (19%), and local recurrence is frequent. Radiation therapy has remained important in treating tumors of the pelvis, skull, and vertebrae that are technically unresectable. Survival (without chemotherapy) is 12.5% at 5 years.

Radiation therapy has played an increasingly important, if not dominant, role in treatment of histiocytic lymphoma (reticulum-cell sarcoma), lymphocytic lymphomas, and plasmacytomas. These tumors are radiosensitive, and true primary lesions are curable by radiation therapy. However, careful evaluation of these lesions will reveal that they are generally widespread and require additional chemotherapy. Ewing's sarcoma has a prompt response to radiation therapy with relief of pain, tumor shrinkage, and healing of bone lesions. Dosages recommended have been in the range of 5000–7000 rads. Recurrence, in Ewings, both locally and widely, has been prompt unless chemotherapy has been used. Single-agent therapy with Actinomycin D, or a combination of Cyclophosphamide, Vincristine, Actinomycin-D, and/ or Adriamycin, has been reported to prevent local recurrence in 51 of 77 patients for periods ranging from 3 to 91 months (9). The combination of radiation and chemotherapy has significantly improved survival data in this highly malignant pediatric tumor and is now considered as standard treatment.

Immunotherapy of bone sarcomas has been prompted by the previously mentioned evidence of a common antigen present in all sarcomas with the association of antibodies in the at-risk population (patients and family contacts). Ivins (10) reports that transfer factor enhances cell-mediated immunity in patients with osteosarcoma. Randomized clinical trials are indicated to adequately evalute the role of immunotherapy.

## SOFT-TISSUE SARCOMAS

This group of tumors is also infrequently diagnosed and is responsible for less than 1% of all malignancies. Because of their rarity these tumors are frequently inadequately and inappropriately treated. Any soft-tissue mass with change in size or consistency warrants incisional biopsy, whether pain is present or not.

Trauma does not appear to be a predisposing factor in soft-tissue sarcomas, although many patients feel otherwise. Soft-tissue sarcomas can arise in scars, after prior radiation, or after long-standing lymphedema. They are also seen in association with Von Recklinghausen's disease, where there is an increase in neurofibrosarcoma.

Primitive mesenchyme has the potential to develop into any type of supportive tissue. For each major type there is one or more corresponding neoplasms: (1) fibrous, fibrosarcoma, (2) adipose, liposarcoma, (3) muscle, rhabdomyosarcoma (four types) and leiomyosarcoma, and (4) vascular, angiosarcoma, and hemangiopericytoma. The frequency of soft-tissue sarcomas varies with age and primary site to some degree. The most common soft-tissue sarcomas in adults are fibrosarcoma and malignant fibrous histiocytoma. There are smaller numbers of leiomyosarcoma, alveolar soft-part sarcoma, rhabdomyosarcoma, synovial sarcoma, angiosarcoma, and undifferentiated sarcoma. In children rhabdomyosarcomas are the most common sarcoma.

Histologic type and grade of tumor (i.e., its inherent degree of malignancy) as well as size have been advocated to define the stage of soft-tissue sarcomas. A retrospective analysis of 702 patients with complete staging reveals a correlation between stage and survival. Prospective studies are now in progress. It is felt by most authorities that these studies will corroborate that the incidence of distant metastases and ultimately survival are related to the histologic grade and size of the primary tumor.

Most soft-tissue sarcomas present as a painless mass with slow growth and are frequently ignored by patients until the tumor assumes rather massive proportions. This location, either superficially in subcutaneous tissue or below the fascia, may be of clinical significance, with the latter tumors having a much poorer prognosis.

Anatomical sites are not usually predictive, but rhabdomysarcomas are frequently found in the proximal extremities of males, liposarcomas are often found in pelvic and shoulder girdles and the retroperitoneum, and synovial sarcomas around the feet, hands, and/or knees. As in the bone sarcomas, hematogenous metastases to the lung are common, but lymph-node metastases do occur in some patients.

Large retroperitoneal and extra-pleural sarcomas can present with severe hypoglycemia, sometimes mimicking a psychotic disorder. This tumor-associated hypoglycemia is almost never caused by secretion of insulin or insulin-like substances. The etiology remains unexplained, although the removal of tumor has been associated with remission of the hypoglycemia.

Adequate staging of soft-tissue sarcomas includes arteriography, gallium scan, bone scan, and whole-chest tomography. Incisional biopsy is the preferable approach, providing that the necrotic tissue is again avoided. With incisional biopsy there is residual gross tumor remaining, but again there is no evidence that this is associated with increased recurrence rates. Although gross tumor often appears encapsulated and well circumscribed, this is merely a pseudocapsule. The sarcomas usually extend along tissue planes into apparently grossly normal structures. Radical surgery is the rule and must include as wide a zone of normal tissue as possible. In sarcomas of the extremities, the surgery must extend to at least one additional uninvolved anatomical structure in both longitudinal and transverse planes. Thus large portions of muscle, neurovascular structure, and bone may be included in the resection. Limb-preserving surgery (11) that avoids amputation has been accomplished using vascular grafts with good local control and long-term survival (3–18 years).

Clinical studies of soft-tissue sarcomas, particularly of the extremities, have been approached by different surgical techniques and varying adjunctive therapy, such as preoperative radiation therapy, immunotherapy, and/or chemotherapy. In a recent review by Simon (12) 54 patients with soft-tissue sarcomas of an extremity treated by surgery alone were evaluated. If patients had adequate surgery (radical local resection, as defined previously, or amputation), the local recurrence rate was only 2%. With inadequate resection, local recurrence is 100%. Interestingly, there appears to be no correlation between histologic type, presence of local recurrence immediate or delayed definitive surgery and the subsequent development of local recurrence or distant metastases. Recurrence was related to adequacy of resection that correlated with the anatomical location of the primary lesion. Distal-extremity lesions had adequate resection, whereas lesions of the proximal extremity and thigh were more likely to have an inadequate resection, with subsequent local recurrence and/or widespread metastases.

Soft-tissue sarcoma of the abdomen, head, and neck is much more difficult to approach, with incomplete resection as a common problem.

The role of radiation therapy has been clouded by the question of varying radiosensitivity of the sarcomas. Many are extremely radioresistant, but there are reports of radiotherapy cure of liposarcomas in the past. Radiation therapy is a primary approach to embryonal rhabdymosarcomas in children.

Lindberg (13) has reported on the use of radiation therapy in addition to surgery in an attempt to preserve a functional limb. They report that of 101 patients (22 trunk, 79 extremities), 71 (11 trunk, 60 extremities) were without evidence of disease at 2 years. They found that local recurrence and metastases was related to both size and grade of the tumor. Patients tolerated doses of radiation as high as 6500 rads in 6.5 weeks fairly well. A functional limb was preserved in 78% of these patients. Technically inoperable sarcomas have been treated with preoperative radiation therapy and subsequent local excision.

Chemotherapy in sarcomas has been evaluated with the same agents as used in bone sarcomas (Adriamycin, high-dose Methotrexate, Vincristine, Actinomycin-D, and DTIC) with response rates of 35–40%. Use as an adjuvant in patients at high risk has begun, but results are certainly too preliminary to determine their value.

Immunotherapy has been utilized in soft-tissue sarcoma with BCG by scarification and/or allogeneic cultured sarcoma cells infected with influenza virus to increase tumor antigenicity. In a nonrandomized study by Townsend (14), recurrence appeared later in patients on BCG immunotherapy. Fifty percent of these patients were disease-free at 42 months, as compared to 25% of untreated control patients. Sinkovics (15) has used immunotherapy in addition to chemotherapy in patients with metastatic disease. He found an increased number of remissions in the combined group as compared to the patients treated with chemotherapy alone. Immunotherapy remains investigational, and these encouraging results are still preliminary communications.

Multimodality treatment of soft-tissue sarcoma has been most successful in the treatment of rhabdomyosarcoma in children, the most common soft-tissue sarcoma in the pediatric population. Rhabdomyosarcoma occurs as a lesion of the head and neck region (especially orbit) in children generally under the age of 10. Botryoidal rhabdomyosarcoma presents as a polypoid mass primarily of the genitourinary tract. Single-agent chemotherapy has been utilized with transient responses for known metastatic disease. Initial studies combined radical surgery plus adjuvant chemotherapy for 1 year (Actinomycin-D and Vincristine) and improved survival rates from past reports and concomitant controls of 50–60% to 90%. The survival rate was still 91% at 3–6 years and was best for patients who had complete removal of the tumor or microscopic residual disease.

Patients with incomplete removal of primary tumor had improved survival rates with the addition of radiation therapy and chemotherapy regimen. Currently chemotherapy is used initially to shrink the bulky primary tumor and to allow less radical surgery. The use of post operative radiation is also being evaluated.

Thus, as in Ewing's sarcoma and osteosarcoma, combined modality treatment has enabled patients to receive less aggressive surgery with preservation and useful function of organs and limbs. The survival at 2 years has been significantly improved from 50% to 90%. These exciting results have made treatment of the sarcomas a multidisciplinary task. Hopefully, this can be applied to other tumors as successfully in the future.

## REFERENCES

1. Morton DL, Eilber FR: Immunologic factors in human sarcomas and melanomas: A rational basis for immunotherapy. Ann Surg 172: 740, 1970.
2. Singh I: Immunologic studies in contacts of osteosarcoma in humans and animals. Nature 265: 541, 1977.
3. Dahlin DC: Bone Tumors, 2nd ed. Charles C Thomas, Springfield, Ill., 1967.
4. Jaffe N: Adjuvant Methotrexate and Citrovorum factor treatment of osteogenic sarcoma. NEJM 291: 944, 1974.
5. Cortes, EP: Amputation and Adriamycin in primary osteosarcoma. NEJM 291: 998, 1974.
6. Jaffe N, Frei E: Osteogenic sarcoma: Advances in treatment. Cancer 26: 351, 1976.
7. Rosen G: Chemotherapy en bloc resection and prosthetic bone replacement in the treatment of osteogenic sarcoma. Cancer 37: 1, 1976.
8. Spanos PK: Pulmonary resection for metastatic osteogenic sarcoma. J Bone Joint Surg 58A: 624, 1976.
9. Jaffe N: The potential of combined modality approaches for the treatment of malignant bone tumors in children. Cancer Treat Rev 2: 33, 1975.

10. Ivins JE: Transfer factor versus combination chemotherapy: A preliminary report. Ann NY Acad Sci 277: 558, 1976.
11. Fortner JG: Limb preserving vascular surgery for malignant tumors of the lower extremities. Arch Surg 112: 391, 1977.
12. Simon M: The management of soft tissue sarcomas of the extremities. J Bone Joint Surg 58A: 317, 1976.
13. Lindberg RD: Soft tissue sarcomas. Curr Prob Cancer 1(5): 4, 1976.
14. Townsend C: Skeletal and soft tissue sarcomas: Treatment with adjuvant immunotherapy. JAMA 236(19): 2187, 1976.
15. Sinkovics JG: Immunotherapy with viral oncolysates for sarcoma (letter). JAMA 237(9): 869, 1977.

# INDEX